High praise for a high drama . . .

"... a masterfully written page-turner of the first order. This is a thriller as compelling as the best that modern fiction has to offer, except that this story is true. I wanted to keep reading. I was sorry when I reached the last page."

Gordon C. Rhea
Author, *The Battle of the Wilderness,*
Winner, Jules and Frances Landry Award

"John Robbins . . . certainly enlightened me on the process of organ transplantation. I was really informed by the stuff he was able to dig up. My hat is off to him. Let's all recycle ourselves. Hell, we recycle everything else—aluminum, plastic—but not organs."

Larry Hagman
Actor
Liver transplant recipient

"Great read! Also a very quick read—I know how the book ends and I reread it anyway because I become absorbed in the human drama every time I open it. *Strings* is the confluence of Barry Hanna, John Lennon, and Will Campbell—all in E.R."

Emory M. Thomas
Author, *Robert E. Lee: A Biography*
Regents Distinguished Professor of History
University of Georgia

"... thoroughly enjoyed the descriptions of characters at MCV—Lee, Mendez, and Carithers. *Strings* captures their personalities beautifully. Robbins is a gifted writer who knows how to paint with words . . ."

Walter Graham
Executive Director
United Network for Organ Sharing (UNOS)

"It can stand alone as a medical thriller; he explains complicated technical issues and makes them exciting, but his spiritual values are what make the book transcendent. This is far more than a well-told tale of a transplant. The man, and the book, are an inspiration."

Nathaniel Tripp
Author, *Father, Soldier, Son:*
Memoir of a Platoon Leader in Vietnam

"*Strings* is written in such a vivid, realistic, and fascinating manner that I could hardly wait to get to the next part."

Jim Beatty
ABC-TV Sports
Track and Field Hall of Fame

"This is a compelling and dramatic story, all the more so because of John Robbins' astonishing grit and courage."

Jeff Stein
Author, *A Murder in Wartime: The Untold Spy Story*
That Changed the Course of the Vietnam War

STRINGS

STRINGS

The Miracle of Life

John B. Robbins

With Forewords by
Gerardo Mendez-Picon, M.D., F.A.C.S.
and
Robert L. Carithers, Jr., M.D.

NORTH STAR PUBLICATIONS
Georgetown, Massachusetts

North Star Publications
P.O. Box 10
Georgetown, MA 01833
(978) 352-9976 • fax (978) 352-5586
http://www.ReadersNdex.com.northstar

Cover design: Salwen Studios, Keene, NH
Editor: John Niendorff

Printed in the United States of America

Publisher's Cataloging-in-Publication

Robbins, John Brawner, 1938-
    Strings : the miracle of life / John Robbins ; with
foregrounds by Robert L. Carithers and Gerardo Mendez-Picon.
– 1st ed.
    p. cm.
    Includes bibliographical references and index.
    ISBN: 1-880823-17-9

    1. Robbins, John Brawner–Health. 2. Liver–
Transplantation. I. Title.

RD546.R63 1998   362.1'975562
                                      QBI98–205

For
Retta

Is it possible to live without feasting on death?
Walker Percy

Contents

Foreword

GERARDO MENDEZ-PICON, M.D., F.A.C.S.

The science of transplantation surgery has made great strides over the past fifteen years. Improvements in the surgical techniques combined with new immunosuppressive drugs have dramatically increased the survival rates of transplant recipients. We have also been able to expand the kinds of medical problems for which transplantation can be an effective treatment. In addition, transplant professionals have been able to increase the age limits of those for whom a transplant can be successful, while at the same time we have decreased the medical complications involved in transplantation and dramatically lowered the morality rate for transplant surgery.

The success of transplantation is best shown by the number of patients waiting for transplant therapy (kidneys, livers, hearts, pancreas, intestines, lungs). From 1988 to 1995, the number of patients waiting for transplants increased by two hundred fifty percent. Unfortunately, during the same period of time, the number of available organs for transplant increased by only eighty percent.

Consequently, the anxiety of the waiting time prior to transplant and the deterioration and possible death of the patient before an organ becomes available have not changed over the years. This is why John Robbins' account of his illness and eventual transplant, as well as his long recovery, are as timely and important today as they were in 1985-87.

John was the first patient in whom we used triple therapy with immunosuppressive drugs. I was very worried that he would not be able to tolerate the new drug regime. His overall state prior to transplant was as close to death as one can get.

The dedication and commitment of each and every member of the transplant team to the patient's well-being are well detailed by John's insightful account. Transplant care professionals have a unique mission. We are driven by numbers and statistics in the analysis of our therapies and their results (such things as percent of rejection episodes during the first year, percent of transplant recipients who survive for five years, survival differences between triple therapy versus induction therapy, etc.). Our daily routine is, on the other hand, the care of people who have both complicated medical problems and unique approaches to life, death, and afterlife.

John Robbins' case is a perfect illustration of the challenges facing both the health-care professional and the patient. He faced a tremendous challenge recovering from both a state of malnutrition and organ failure (his liver function before surgery was so bad, it was close to non-existent). It was the race of his life.

In most surgical events, when surgery is completed successfully, ninety percent of the problems which the patient faces are over. In transplant surgery the percentages are reversed. When the last skin stitch is placed, ninety percent of potential complications lie ahead.

When we finished John's surgery, he started his race, with our transplant staff as the cheering crowd, helping him along by our daily monitoring and therapeutic changes. We could help him, but we could not run for him. He had to do the tough part alone.

The race to the finish line in a transplant recipient is an interesting one. When you cross the line, you have fully recovered and you feel the great satisfaction of regaining your sense of well-being. In contrast, in a road race, especially a marathon, when you finish, you reach the highest point of exhaustion. I assure you that in both races, each step has to be fought equally hard, and it gets harder the closer you are to the finish line.

GERARDO MENDEZ-PICON, M.D., F.A.C.S.

Vascular and General Surgery
Surgical Director, Kidney Transplant Program
Henrico Doctors' Hospital
Richmond, Virginia

Foreword

ROBERT L. CARITHERS, JR., M.D.

This is an exciting and important book. John Robbins has captured both the frustration and the miracle of modern transplantation from a unique perspective—that of a critically ill patient who survived a liver transplant. As he so poignantly describes, John literally walked through the valley of the shadow of death before his transplant. Miraculously, he survived the operation and has recovered to the point that he has run marathons and written a book—two feats many of us never will accomplish! John's story is truly a testament to the invincibility of the human spirit.

John does a beautiful job of capturing the agony, abandonment, and mistrust many patients and their families feel during the long wait for a donor organ. As he describes, it is very easy for even the most rational families to believe that they have been abandoned and lied to, not only by the system but also by health-care professionals they have trusted, in whose care they have placed their lives. Because of an increasing shortage of donor organs, this frustration is even more acute for patients currently waiting for liver, heart, lung, kidney, or pancreas transplants.

At the same time, John very skillfully describes the remarkable teamwork which must occur for an organ transplant to be successful. The drama that he outlines goes on daily in transplant centers, unbeknownst to most of the public. Furthermore, he dramatically captures the quiet dedication of the many people—the procurement team, the pilots, the many wonderful nurses, the technicians, and the highly skilled surgeons—who make transplantation possible. This sense of dedication and teamwork should be a source of deep reassurance to any person or family considering organ donation.

Last but not least, John shows us how important the support of friends, family, and compassionate health-care professionals is to the recovery from the major surgery required for most transplant operations. Without such support, recovery is difficult, if not impossible. With such support, miracles can happen even under the most difficult circumstances. It is this human face of transplantation which John has so beautifully captured in this book.

Strings should be an inspiration to many. To patients, to families, to potential donors and their families, and even to health-care professionals who may have become burned out with the frustrations associated with transplantation. We all need to remember how miraculous transplantation is and how it can so profoundly affect so many lives. This book reminds us how blessed we are to have such an opportunity to start new cycles of life every day.

ROBERT L. CARITHERS, JR., M.D.

Professor of Medicine
Medical Director of Liver Transplant Programs
University of Washington, Seattle, Washington

Strings

Beginnings

The path exists, but not the man on it.
Vissudhimagga

Jay always said this is the way it would end, Joan thinks to herself as she stands at my bedside at Mary Washington Hospital in Fredericksburg, Virginia. Family and close friends gather at the hospital as my three-year fight draws to its inevitable conclusion. I am hours from death, in an hepatic coma in the intensive care unit. My liver has failed. My sister, Retta, leaves my bedside to tell our friend Janet Payne, "You'd better go in now and see John, if . . . ." She doesn't finish; it isn't necessary. Janet understands.

Retta leaves Janet and calls my best friend from college days, Ray Wallace, to tell him the news. Ray in turn activates a network of old college acquaintances who had pulled together in an effort to save my life. Hearing the news of the coma, Nell Drew, wife of one of my college classmates, sighs quietly, "Well, we did all we could, didn't we, Ray?"

"Yes, Nell, we did," Ray observes sadly, but then vents his anger. "Those bastards at MCV just didn't get him the liver in time, and now it's too late."

Several hours later, as Joan stands her turn in the death-watch in the ICU, Valerie Sherman, a critical care nurse in the ICU, enters the room quietly and whispers to Joan, who is staring intently at my comatose body, "There's a call from MCV for anyone in the family."

Joan hurries from the room, answers the telephone, and slides to the floor as she hears: "We're moving John to Richmond. We think we've found a liver." The steady, calm voice of Ann Reid Priest, clinical nurse specialist who handles the logistics of liver transplants at the Medical College of Virginia, brings the only glimmer of hope to the sad day. The

1

call begins thirty-six hours of almost perpetual motion. First it sets into action a complex logistical effort to get a patient, a donated organ, and a transplant team all coordinated in one spot under demanding time constraints. The arrangements begin a multifaceted story of transplant.

Strings is a tale—

- of dramatic events that cheat death;
- of modern medicine at its best;
- of hope, prayer, miracle after miracle, and odds defied and overcome;
- of family and friends whose lives are profoundly affected by the transplant process;
- of a group of extraordinary professionals who make up the liver transplant team at the Medical College of Virginia.

The MCV team was an amazingly diverse and talented group. It included an explosive, bearded, demanding, egocentric Spanish surgeon who is a member of the ACLU; an internist who is both a scientist and a humanist English major and who can keep surgeons, psychologists, psychiatrists, social workers, chaplains, dieticians, nurses, patients, and families all pulling together; an unusually caring, thoughtful clinical nurse specialist who is deeply proud of her profession and ramrods the program with the iron hand of a marine drill sergeant while touching the patients with the gentle hand of a nurturing mother; a dietician who cares for patients far beyond the call of duty; a psychologist who comforts and understands the unique mental strains of transplant and battles the surgeon for the patient's well-being; and an Episcopalian intern and counselor in the hospital chaplain's office who explains Buddhism to the transplant team.

Most of all *Strings* is a personal story, a story of personal quest. The experience called upon me to examine life more intensely than ever before and provided, in a strange way, a rare opportunity for me to take charge of my own destiny.

The years from the onset of my liver disease to the transplant itself gave me a great deal of time to wonder about creation, with its beginning and end, with its birth, death, and possibility of rebirth. It became a poignant time for me, someone who had earlier uprooted his middle-class existence and wandered the jungles of Southeast Asia as a

Buddhist monk, searching for meaning. End-stage liver disease, resulting from hepatitis B I contracted nine years earlier in India, suddenly and dramatically transformed my search from the theoretical to the real. For three years, I stared daily at death. I talked about it often. The talking made it real. I came to understand that separating life from death or beginning from end is a learned reaction that does not flow from the nature of things as they truly are.

My quest for understanding has been lifelong. As a schoolboy, I thrilled to questing in all forms, particularly to Henry David Thoreau's life at Walden and his philosophy in "Civil Disobedience." I often felt I heard a different drummer and must disobey what I thought was wrong. From grammar school to young adulthood there were wrongs to be righted, causes to be supported. As I grew older and accumulated more experience, I saw more to questing than simply a good and thrilling story; a spiritual dimension expanded its meaning for me. At first, I quite naturally turned to Christianity and to Western philosophy to explore beyond the Episcopalian ritual of my youth. Later the writings of the American transcendentalists, French *philosophes*, and existentialists opened new avenues. Finally Eastern, particularly Buddhist, thought fueled my quest.

I always identified with the Don Quixotes of the world and felt that we are called to tilt at windmills, believing this effort is not futile, but noble. Conversely, I accepted the cosmic insignificance of my own existence. What really makes any difference? Of what importance is my own being? With Camus' Outsider, I "laid . . . my heart open to the benign indifference of the universe." And with the Taoists, I intuitively understood that "it is just because one has no use for life that one is wiser than the man who values life." Experience with Eastern thought and languages taught me that to acknowledge the indifference of the universe and the valuelessness of life is not nihilistic, but hopeful and positive. Accepting death and fighting for life are not opposites. They only appear opposite to undeveloped minds. However, watching me fight for life in a way that appeared to involve my accepting death confused family, friends, and most of all, doctors. At times it confused even me.

○

"When you understand the teaching that 'the path exists, but not the man on the path,' you will understand Buddhism and the East." Tan Mutti, a 78-year-old Chinese-Thai monk, who had spent nineteen years alone in a cave, told me at the conclusion of one of our frequent conversations at Suan Mok, a forest monastery in the Southern Thai jungle.

The inscrutable East, I thought to myself, *being mysterious for the sake of seeming wise. Surely this makes no sense.* "What do you mean?" I protested. "What's the answer?"

"If you seek an answer, you'll never understand," he replied gently.

I dropped the subject, realizing I would never get anywhere and certainly would never understand. After all, I reasoned, if he couldn't explain the answer, the statement obviously had no real meaning. I went back to my small hut in the jungle, troubled and feeling blocked. I gave up trying to reason and thought to myself, *If that's what it takes to understand this world, I'm not going to make it. I just don't think I have to do it the way Tan Mutti tells me.*

I went merrily on my own way, drawing strength from my favorite Zen tale, in which a student approached a renowned master and asked to be enlightened. The wise old man replied that he could not teach enlightenment because only two things could result from such an attempt. First, the student might misinterpret the lesson and make the teacher look foolish. Second, since the master's knowledge was his own and could never be anyone else's, he could never teach "enlightenment." As both possibilities were unsatisfactory, he dismissed the student.

An incident in my own life made this tale real. One day, I asked my teacher and abbot, the wise old Buddhist monk Buddhadasa, to explain a subtle point of Buddhist metaphysics, namely the *patticcasamuppada,* or theory of dependent origination, by which Buddhists explain the circular nature of the world. He smiled and answered. I took notes, went back to my hut, analyzed, reasoned, memorized, dissected and used my intellect with great precision. I was sure I could write answers, handle the material in graduate school seminar parlance, lecture on the subject, and sound quite "intellectual" and knowledgeable. Several months later Buddhadasa asked me casually if I understood *patticcasamuppada.*

"Of course," I replied proudly and proceeded to give my best seminar-style answer to the master.

"But do you understand it?" he persisted after my reply.

"No." I had to admit quietly that I didn't understand all I knew.

"*Mai pen rai, banya yang mai paw*. Don't worry, your wisdom is not yet fully developed," he said.

Although momentarily comforted, I still wondered how wisdom is developed. After all, I had an earned doctorate, had spent most of the first thirty-five years of my life in intellectual environments, and still felt I was not among the wise. I questioned my meditation masters, "How do we obtain wisdom and how do we know what it is?"

"It comes when you need it."

My earlier years spent searching for a meditation teacher had brought a strikingly similar response. "You will find your teacher when you need him."

During our first conversations, when Tan Mutti observed me writing down his words, he cautioned, "Don't write. Throw away your notes and your books. Your Western mind, though well-trained, is too sticky. If you understand what I say or what you read, then when you need it, it will be there."

I put away my pencil and listened. In the process I learned to avoid the Western trap of making the East seem too simple. Often Eastern philosophy appeals to Westerners because it seems to be saying, "Sit back, wait for that moment of enlightenment, and then you will know." I must admit that this has a certain attraction, but it can lead one to overlook the absolute necessity of preparing the way. Wisdom is a subtle interplay of action/experience and thought. One must be reflective and possess the mental discipline to understand one's experience. Many have experiences; few understand them. I observed hundreds of young people "on the road" in the sixties and seventies who were having wonderful experiences, but who, at the same time, lacked the mental discipline to understand what they were experiencing or feeling.

Action must always be accompanied by thought. The two cannot be separated. Acting and thinking, health and sickness, life and death, doctor and patient are one and the same thing. We seem unable to grasp this unity because of a commitment to dualism. The heart of the sixties' experience—from the writings of Castaneda, Hesse, Alpert, and Kesey to rock music, drugs, and Eastern mysticism—challenged this assumption. I spent a lot of time and effort trying to "know" and to "feel" unity, because I was taught that thought and feeling, mind and emotion, reason and intuition, the "observer and the observed"—to borrow the words of J. Krishnamurti—were mutually exclusive or at best did not operate together. A catastrophic illness that forced me to live for a long time dealing with death led to a real understanding that life and death, thought and action, thought and feeling are not so different after all. Philosophies without action are only words. Action without heart is only movement.

Part I

LIFE

The unexamined life is not worth living.
— Socrates

The unlived life is not worth examining.
— Kant

1

Shirt and Strings

For either killing or creating may be a crime
punishable by death and the death always comes by
the criminal's own hand and every man is a suicide.
If a man knew how to live he would never die.

Robert Penn Warren, *All the King's Men*

God, it's foggy. Fog is everywhere. I'm inside, aren't I? Yes, I think I am . . . what's happening? I'm all bloody.

The fog lifts slowly and reality returns. Rushing from the eleventh floor of the Asia Apartments in the Rajatevi section of Bangkok to the hospital after another in a succession of internal bleeding incidents is only a dim memory. I hear Thai sounds swimming in my ears. I speak Thai fluently, but the words are jumbled. Tired of struggling and determined to surrender to my fate peacefully, I am firm in my resolve to die. After a series of experiences like this, I understand the inevitable outcome. Lying in the emergency room, I am not denying death, but rather feeling a little excitement at experiencing the unknown.

It is August 20, 1984—a month and eight days before my 46th birthday, my fifth trip to the hospital since it all began in October 1983. By now I know the routine pretty well. I spent hours since my last trip to the hospital researching both the function of the liver and its diseases. I learned, according to my medical dictionary, that the liver, "produces bile [which aids in the digestion of fats and performs a vital function of detoxification of poisons in the body], converts most sugars into glycogen [which fuels the muscles], and it is essential to life." In a way,

9

the liver is a combination Betty Ford Center and a Health Spa, as it both clears the body of toxins and converts food and vitamins into muscle and energy. It is, thus, necessary for almost all physical and mental functions. When a liver becomes scarred (cirrhotic) and cannot perform its basic functions, death results. In my case, the liver became cirrhotic from viral hepatitis B I had suffered nine years previously in India. Because the blood cannot flow freely through a cirrhotic liver, the result is hypertension (high pressure) in the portal vein (one of the two major blood supplies to the liver). Blood then attempts to return to the heart by alternative means, creating varices (distended vessels in the lining of the esophagus) and major bleeding. When the sickness reaches this endstage, time to live is measured in months, certainly no longer than a year.

The reoccurring attacks happen suddenly: the feeling of nausea, the dryness in the throat, the headache, the absolute and utter fatigue, the inability to walk without bouncing off the walls, the trips to the bathroom, vomiting the thick black venous blood. It's variceal bleeding again. The scars in my liver are causing the blood vessels in my esophagus to burst.

I ask myself, *How can it happen again?* Reality takes hold. *Why am I surprised? It's all making more sense now. Oh yes, it's clear now. My life is slipping away quickly. Oh good, the fog is lifting. It's over. It must certainly be a matter of minutes now. I will just sit back, relax, and see what else I can learn. Death is life's final lesson. After all, death is the last thing I have to experience.*

Events of my life rush through me in a stream of consciousness: a happy childhood; my education at Hampden-Sydney College and Rice University; teaching at the University of North Carolina-Charlotte in one of the most exciting ten years in the history of American education; political activism; the war; peace; music; books; wandering the world; crossing the Asian continent twice by land; exploring Europe and the British Isles; drinking tea with the Bedouins; climbing mountains in Southeast Asia; experiencing the thrill of whitewater canoeing in Canada; three years as a Buddhist monk; family, students, colleagues, and friends strung around the world in countries on five continents; reading many of the world's great books; seeing for myself most of the world's art treasures and monuments; knowing the excitement of ideas and the joy of friends. So much passes in front of me now so quickly.

Sure it shouldn't end, but it's time. My thoughts turn to Thoreau, who believed that most men fear dying because, when it came time to die, they realized they had not lived. *Surely he wasn't writing about me,* I comforted myself.

The Emergency Room is busy with activity. Young interns and medical students are running about, earnestly carrying out their assigned tasks. I know everyone is tense. The nurses and doctors are speaking freely. "Quiet," I hear one of them caution the other in Thai. "He speaks Thai."

Many on the staff know me pretty well by now. Westerners don't often come to the Emergency Room at the Thai government hospital named for King Rama V, Chulalongkorn.

In goes one IV for glucose and then another for transfusions. I'm spinning quickly and sliding into unconsciousness. Perhaps I will bleed to death. I know the procedure by now: the tube is inserted through the nose and an iced solution follows to cool the bleeding area, much as one might use cold water to stop the bleeding on a cut finger. If that fails, next comes the esophageal balloon, a device inserted through the nose into the esophagus and inflated to act as a compress on the bleeding. It hurts. The last resort is emergency surgery that, I hear them say, I probably can't survive. No matter; I'm resigned. I will accept my impermanence and not make karma for the future. I am only slightly angry because I had hoped to die peacefully, in quieter circumstances, so I could focus more clearly on my life and death and see what the cycle had to teach me before it started all over again.

I begin to reassure myself. *It's time. Give up. I must keep my promise to go calmly. Work is no longer possible. It's clear I can't earn a living. I have no insurance and can never return to America, so what's the use? With this bleed my life is, in effect, over. It's happened. Let it be. This too shall pass.*

Suddenly my calming attempt is shattered. *What's happening?* I wonder. Someone is moving a complicated-looking machine toward me. The Thai is unintelligible.

Wait . . . what's this? The nurse has scissors in her hand. What are they going to do? Oh no, they're going to cut off my shirt to hook something else to me.

I look down. My shirt is soaked in blood, but through the blood I see one of my prized possessions, something I brought with me the last time

I came to Thailand from North Carolina—my "1982 Carolina No. 1" T-shirt celebrating the Michael Jordan shot that gave the 'Heels the NCAA national title.

Gad, they can't cut it off. I can never get another one. It's priceless, I think to myself. I yell out as loudly as the situation allows: "*Ham taat sua! Ham taat sua*! Don't cut my shirt!"

In the midst of my yelling, a chilling thought sweeps over me. *The Thai word for shirt is "sua," but it is also the Thai word for "mat" and "tiger." The only difference is tones. Let's see, high tone is used for "tiger," falling tone for "shirt," and low tone for"mat"—or is it the other way around? Damn, I can't remember. I must try something, but with all these tubes in me, am I getting it right? Or am I saying, "Don't cut the tiger?" Perhaps they think I'm delirious or crazy. They don't understand.*

"*Ham taat sua, ham taat sua*. Don't cut my shirt, don't cut my shirt." At that moment I hear my friend Noui saying (excitedly for a Thai), ". . . he loves that shirt. It's something about some basketball game. It's a sport in America and his state is proud of it or something like that. Do you have to cut it off?"

"No! We'll try to take it over his head and then you can clean it up," responds one of the obliging Thais.

The whole process stops while my shirt is saved. I stare at the shirt as Noui retrieves it from the nurses and remind myself, *Perhaps I'm not yet ready to die. Maybe one more fight might be worth the effort.*

o

I was in the emergency room at Chulalongkorn Hospital in Bangkok that night because I was an American expatriate living in Asia. I had originally left the United States in 1974 because I often felt trapped between the "establishment" and the "counterculture." As a member of the silent fifties, I, like my generational counterparts, had found admission to university and access to good jobs fairly easily. We had risen in our chosen professions rapidly. For example, I finished my Ph.D. before I was 26 and earned tenure before 30. Early success gave me—and many in my generation—time to think. "We were kind of mindlessly goal-oriented," I told a reporter from the Charlotte *News* who asked why I had surrendered tenure, "and we decided on careers without really wondering if that's what we wanted. Then you get in your mid-thirties and you wonder. . . . you grow up and then you realize—all I am is older, the questions are still there. . . . You're asking the same questions, but this time you understand what they mean."

I went to meditation classes, sensitivity-training retreats, experimented with the drugs of the Leary generation, and followed rock bands. In short, I did all the things that characterized those heady times of peace, love, and rock and roll. Instinctively, I understood the ephemeral nature of these experiences and sought something more, something lasting.

A recent divorce gave me the freedom to wander, so I left both my career and country because I felt I needed time and perspective to look at my life. My quest took me from Charlotte to Canada for whitewater canoeing; to London, where I began a journey overland to New Delhi. I arrived in the Indian city debilitated with hepatitis. I went to Bangkok to recuperate, fell in love with the Thais and Asia. It seemed like a good place to stop, so I got a job at a Thai university.

My interest in Eastern thought, stimulated by my earlier reading of transcendentalism and existentialism, led me to a Buddhist monastery where I practiced meditation while living the life of a Buddhist monk for three years. In those years I learned patience, realized that I didn't know everything, and learned not to hate and be angry. I had been out of the United States for almost eight years, then at the end of 1981, I returned. But I missed Thailand and life in a Buddhist country. After consulting with my cousin, who at the time was head of the International Division of North Carolina National Bank (now NationsBank), I returned to Thailand in 1983 to open a consulting and importing-exporting business. I was just getting started when hepatitis from my previous trip to India caught up with me.

o

My Thai business partner, Theera, assumed the responsibility of relaying information about my medical condition to my family and friends in the United States. After this latest attack, he called my sister in Fredericksburg. "Retta, John thinks you might want to know that he's bleeding again and in the hospital. But don't worry. He's alive and okay now." His calls, coming with a kind of monotonous regularity, no longer reassured her.

She, in turn, called our brother, Jay, who is a physician. "John's in the hospital again. What should we do?"

"There's not much we can do. This is a very serious situation, and John's prognosis is virtually hopeless."

This answer troubled Retta. She was angry because Jay acted like a doctor, not a brother. "I wish we could get him to come home," she replied. "I can take care of him until he recovers."

"Retta, he's not going to recover . . . ever."

While my family fretted and called both Theera and my doctor, Sommai Vilairattana, I remained in critical condition in the hospital, deciding I would like to live a little while longer. Noui washed my Carolina shirt carefully and came to the hospital to tell me it was okay. I lay in a ward for three days while seconds passed like hours, minutes like weeks, hours like months. I tried to meditate: *Breathe in and know that I am breathing in; breathe out and know that I am breathing out; breaths get longer and longer . . . .*

I repeated the *Maranassati* or "Mindfulness of Death Meditation":

Jaradhammohi Jaram, Anatitio,
["I am of the nature to decay; I have not gone beyond decay,"]
Byadhidahammohi Byadhim Anatitio,
["I am of the nature to sicken; I have not gone beyond sickness"]
Maranadhammohi Maranam Anatitio,
["I am of the nature to die; I have not gone beyond death."]

This had been part of my daily meditations at 4 a.m. for almost three years. But those meditations didn't shorten the time the tubes were in me. I was not centered properly. The ego raged and I worried about death. I pleaded with myself. *Death would be better than this. Let me die. It's not worth the fight. I seem to get to the edge of death and then step back. It's such a close step, let me take it.* But I didn't die; I couldn't take that step.

Despite another bleeding episode in the hospital two days later, the therapy eventually worked. The treatment—which consisted of sclerotherapy (a process in which a tube is inserted into the esophagus and medicine is injected to permanently harden the bleeding point to stop further hemorrhaging), glucose, and massive blood transfusion to rebuild my strength—saved my life once again. Several other things were at work simultaneously during this period. I still had some fight left; I centered myself; and, after looking at death so closely in a heightened sense of reality, I decided life was the better choice. A lot of credit, of course, goes to my friends who rallied around me. Ten days later I left Chulalongkorn University Hospital, a little unsteady but still breathing.

Spending extended periods on the critical list had become a routine part of my existence for over a year and half since the time I first collapsed outside of class one evening while teaching English as a Second Language at the American University Alumni Language Center in Bangkok.

"Noui," I said, after he had settled me in the apartment, "I'm going back to America, but only for a rest, and then I'll come back. You stay in my apartment and watch things for me while I am gone. I will be back, I promise. I want to live in Thailand. Go to the wat [monastery], feed nine monks for me on my birthday, and behave yourself. I'll be back."

"You should stay in America and let the doctors take care of you. They are better than the ones in Thailand," he counseled.

"I can't stay in America, Noui, because I don't have any money." I reminded him that I was almost out of funds and therefore could not afford medical care in the United States. He didn't understand that the health care system in a country as rich as America could place a premium on money. He didn't believe me.

After a series of international calls, cabled money, and quick reservations, I left for the United States a little more than a year after I had returned to live permanently in Thailand. *I'll be back. I'll be back,* I promised myself.

"See you soon," I assured my Thai friends when I showed my passport and entered the departure area at Don Muang, Bangkok's International Airport. In fact, I had little choice but to keep my promise to return. I could not afford to stay in America. Since I worked abroad, I had no medical insurance in the United States and, furthermore, could not get any. Since I could afford to pay for medical care in Thailand, returning to Asia seemed the only option I had. I was priced out of my native land.

O

I learned, much to my dismay, that two months' rest in America didn't solve the problem. On a New Year's Eve night, less than a month after I returned to Thailand, it happened again. Bleeding put me in the hospital. I greeted 1985 with tubes in my nose, with virtual nonstop medical care. Once again this procedure stopped the bleeding and sclerotherapy worked to harden the bleeding point. But I bled again in the summer as the varices kept progressing lower and lower along the esophageal tract, which made it increasingly difficult for the doctors to stem the bleeding with sclerotherapy. Each bleed brought me close to death, but the treatment continued to work.

The bleeding episodes reached their climax on October 19, 1985. I couldn't remember how it began that night. All I knew is that I looked up in great pain and recognized that a serious situation was unfolding around me.

O

Amidst the haze of confusion and pain, I see Noui moving toward me with a piece of string. As he draws closer, I recognize its orange color and its distinctive knots. It is a *sai sila*, a cotton string tied around the wrist to represent a connection with the Sangha, the followers of the Buddha. Some Thais wear the string (sometimes more than one) for protection, much as, in the Christian tradition, a Roman Catholic might wear a St. Christopher's medal. Tonight Noui is using this *sai sila* as a kind of Buddhist last rite. The doctors tell him I am dying. He takes one look at me and agrees. Since he's been through this with me many times before, he understands the situation well. He moves quietly toward me and says, "This is from the monks at my wat. It is very special," and he ties it around my right wrist. An hour later, after watching me go from yellow to a sickening kind of grey, he ties yet another around my left wrist.

It must really be near now, I think.

It's a little over a year since the incident with the shirt and three weeks after my 47th birthday. I am not able to thank Noui for the strings, or even smile, because the esophageal balloon inflated in an attempt to stop the bleeding inside my esophagus is anchored by wire to a mask that covers my face. My head is throbbing and I ache all over. This is clearly my worst bleeding incident. I know I will be dead in a matter of hours. I wish once again, as I had a year ago, that I might see Ret, but I know I am not going to last that long.

I look at my strings and know they tie me to family and friends. I try to accept things as they are, seeking a special understanding that allows me to remain detached from the struggle—in other words, to fight without fighting. As a result, struggling never consciously crosses my mind. The strength to fight for life can only come to one who remains detached from the fight and unconcerned with the outcome. I understand instinctively that I can truly fight only as long as I am unaware of the struggle. My situation is like breath itself. I do not make a conscious choice to breathe. In the same manner, I cannot make any deliberate choice to fight. Rational analysis is useless. Thought doesn't help. It can't on such occasions.

I recall sitting for hour upon hour in mindfulness-of-breath meditation in the jungle or at the seaside where I first glimpsed the mystery of effortless effort. I know I need it now. My life depends on my success in mastering this concept—it is no longer a question of theory. I reach, without reaching, for "my beginner's mind," in which "all things are possible." Survival clearly dictates acceptance without thought, a child's unquestioning love and trust. I seek, without seeking, a kind of equanimity and acceptance, an acceptance that transcends resignation. I know there is a subtle and powerful difference between acceptance and resignation. I understand that my life sways in the delicate balance inherent in that recognition.

o

Several days later, a young Thai doctor appeared in my room. "Mr. Robbins, I am Dr. Chanvit, a surgeon on the staff of the medical school." This doctor spoke English better than I. He had, like so many upper-class Thais, been exclusively educated abroad. From elementary-school days through post-medical school training, he had studied in England. Chanvit Tanphiphat, Associate Professor of Surgery, was my first introduction to surgeons in Thailand. "East is East, and West is West, and never the twain shall meet," wrote Rudyard Kipling. Perhaps he never met a surgeon. They're all alike: surgery is the only way to fix any medical problem.

Dr. Chanvit presented me with a new twist in my medical history: choosing between options when two doctors advised differing courses of treatment. Dr. Sommai wanted to continue with sclerotherapy, while Dr. Chanvit opted for a surgical solution. The young surgeon explained to me, "Sclerotherapy is simply not doing the job and if you bleed again they may not be able to stop it by irrigation, the balloon, or sclerotherapy.* Surgery under these conditions is very risky, with only about a five percent chance of survival. Yet, I recommend the surgical procedure known as a portacaval shunt, which allows the blood flowing through the portal vein, one of the major blood vessels leading into the liver, to bypass the organ and thereby reduce the hypertension [pressure] that is causing your blood vessels to burst and bleed. I don't want to have to do surgery on you under emergency conditions, because I am concerned that it cannot be done. Dr. Sommai doesn't understand the gravity of this kind of surgery under emergency situations."

"Well, Doctor, this is a little sudden and I have been with Dr. Sommai over a year now. I just can't make a sudden change. I will have to think it over. What are the risks of the surgery?"

"If we undertake an intensive program to prepare you, the chances of survival are reasonably good," he replied rather matter-of-factly. "It is, of course, not a cure for your liver disease, though it may allow you to live longer with the hepatitis under control. There are no certainties."

"Perhaps you and Dr. Sommai could talk again and consult with my brother. Please call him in America. Dr. Sommai has his number," I answered, as a way of deciding not to decide at the moment.

Dr. Sommai was next in to see me. "American doctors are not doing that surgery anymore. Ask your brother. Its implications are rather

---

* To summarize these three procedures: Irrigation involves inserting a tube and a cold solution into the esophagus to cool the area in an attempt to stem bleeding. The balloon involves inserting and inflating a tube into the esophagus to act as a compress to stop the bleeding. Sclerotherapy is a process in which a tube is inserted in the esophagus, and then a medicine is injected to permanently harden the bleeding point in hopes of preventing future bleeding. Dr. Sommai treated me with sclerotherapy on five separate occasions, from July 1984 to September 1985. The treatment has been used successfully in many cases, but did not work for me, as bleeding points kept breaking out in fresh areas of the esophagus, progressively closer to the stomach.

dangerous and, post-operatively, it may hasten the decline of your liver function. Most of the foreign doctors I consult with are not doing this type of surgery anymore, either," he concluded, suggesting that citing what was done abroad would win the argument with me.

Unfortunately, I did not recognize the full implications of his warning. For example, a portacaval shunt means the liver does not get an adequate blood flow, which prevents it from functioning to its normal capacity. The result often compromises liver function, causing a build-up of various noxious substances, such as ammonia, in the bloodstream. These substances can, in turn, adversely affect the brain and cause confusion, trembling, and malaise after the procedure. Another way of putting it: the person is getting slowly poisoned. At the time, however, unaware of that daunting possibility, I simply said, "Well, I just don't know what to do. Let me think about it."

"Fine," he replied. "I will talk to Dr. Chanvit and with your brother, who asked me to take care of you."

After a year and a half of bimonthly visits and five trips to Chula-longkorn Hospital, I had spent a lot of time with Dr. Sommai, who had become an integral part of my life. Chairman of the Department of Gastroenterology and president of the Gastroenterological Society of Thailand, he gave me, a foreigner and a clinic patient, his time gener-ously and unselfishly. We talked often about Buddhism and about my teacher, Buddhadasa Bhikku. The doctor had a Buddhist altar and a picture of the King of Thailand in his office. He was proud of his background as the son of an upcountry rice farmer. Like all Thais he valued family. When my brother wrote him about my treatment, Dr. Sommai took most seriously the charge from a fellow doctor to care for his younger brother. I heard him explain one day to his nurse, "We must find him the right room; his older brother, a doctor, has placed him in my care."

He was always cheerful and confident; we never talked about death. Thai doctors are not absorbed with a sometimes mindless attempt to extend life beyond all hope. Death is not the great tragedy it is in the West. Death is accepted more gracefully, because the model of Thai medical behavior is not male and Western. Death is not seen as something that defeats the efforts of the doctor. Death is not final. Most Buddhist Asians do not see life and death in macho terms of win or lose. As a result they tend to deal with death much more comfortably and naturally than do their Western counterparts. They see it for what it is, an inevitable part of the life process. It is not that Asians are callous; it is rather that they have a different view of life that Westerners often misunderstand. They revere life and their families. Death, however, is not an end, but a transition. They lack a Western sense of guilt.

Although I was a clinic patient rather than a private patient, Dr. Sommai continued to give unselfishly of his time throughout the year and a half he treated me. Noui often called him in the middle of the night, and he came to the hospital time and time again to see me. He was a healer and a doctor—not a businessman. We never discussed money except on one amazing occasion.

"Dr. Sommai, should I go home to the United States for treatment?"

"Well, I don't think you'll find a better doctor, though possibly a doctor in Germany may be better than I am. You might, however, find a doctor in a large American medical center who does nothing but sclerotherapy. But you would then face two problems. First, would they accept you as a patient? And second, you don't have insurance, and in your country they will probably not take care of you without money. I'll take care of you."

He spoke the truth. I was not even a citizen in this, what we euphemistically call a Third World country, and a doctor committed himself and his institution to my care. The conversation stuck in my consciousness. I always recall it when I hear people say how lucky we are to be Americans.

On Thursday, the 24th of October, Dr. Sommai visited again and reported that he and Dr. Chanvit had reached a tentative agreement. Dr. Sommai would continue with sclerotherapy and schedule an exam and treatment on the 31st. If I had another bleeding attack after that, Sommai would agree to the surgery.

On Friday, Noui arrived to take care of me for the weekend—until Monday when I would probably be discharged from the hospital. But Saturday morning another incident of variceal bleeding interrupted my recovery. This was the tenth major bleeding incident since it all began in October 1983. I knew from my research into liver disease that this was a high number and that my chance of surviving another major bleed was slim. (Few people survive as many as five major incidents of variceal bleeding.) I had already spent a total of forty-seven days in the hospital before this stay, which had so far added another eight days to my total, with no end in sight. This new bleed on Saturday morning, only one week from the bleed that brought me to the brink of death, meant I could no longer postpone the fateful decision about surgery. Attacks were coming days—rather than weeks—apart.

In the afternoon, I began the torturous process of figuring out what do to. I reviewed my notebook in which I had been keeping a brief summary of medical appointments, treatments, and trips to the Emergency Room and hospital. It ran to ten pages. I took stock of my situation. I knew I had to make my decision alone. *Of course, I said to myself, I have to decide by myself. Who else can make a decision affecting my own life and death?*

I began yet another of my many internal dialogues in which I debated the pros and cons of life and death. I recalled a philosophy that I had scribbled in my diary suggested by a Bob Dylan song. Essentially Dylan seemed to be saying that no one else knows better than you, you're only doing what you're meant to be doing, and it doesn't matter anyway. It was probably as good a sense of Buddhist philosophy as I had read anywhere, although I'm not sure Dylan thought of it as such.

I understood his philosophy not as a statement of resignation and pessimism, but rather as a positive affirmation of life—one that made my decision easier. Another factor that made my decision easier was that I was lying in a hospital in Bangkok, halfway around the world from childhood attachments and family. Family and attachment are a double-edged sword. On one side, they are extremely confining when you are trying to live your own life, but, on the other side, they are extraordinarily supportive when you are facing the sometimes difficult consequences brought on by your choices.

Finally, my decision came rather easily. After cursing my fate—*Why can't I just live or die like everyone else? Why do I have to make a choice?*—I reasoned that the recurring attacks made me feel like a prisoner in Bangkok. I felt trapped, and concluded that life like this was not worth living. I called out to no one in particular, "I am going to have the portacaval shunt." I relaxed.

Dr. Chanvit came to see me on Sunday. He told me that Dr. Sommai had concurred in the wisdom of the surgery in light of the Saturday morning bleed. Everyone was in accord. Dr. Sommai wrote orders for therapy to strengthen me for the surgery. With the decision made, the only thing ahead of me was, of course, the surgery itself—which was highly risky. It was scheduled for November 8, and that seemed lifetimes away.

Noui looked troubled when he came to see me in the afternoon. "Why doesn't your family love you? *Nong chai* [younger brother] is in the hospital and your elder brother and sister are not here. What's wrong?" Noui had been rallying all of his friends to visit me at the hospital, but just couldn't understand why my brother and sister were not there with me.

"Noui, they love me, but they work and it's a very long distance, halfway around the world, to come here. They just can't leave work and fly so far to be with me." I could tell my words made no impression. As an Asian, he would never understand nursing homes, retirement communities, and hospital stays without family. That evening, however, a beaming Noui came to tell me Ret would arrive in Bangkok at 8:30 p.m. on the Tuesday before the surgery on Friday. He was relieved that I hadn't been forgotten!

Retta arrived on a beautiful, warm, tropical Bangkok evening. A business associate of mine met her and brought her to the hospital. She was a little taken aback by the scene she found. Expecting a somber, drab hospital room, she entered the hospital compound through a courtyard with verdant, fragrant shrubbery, climbed the steps to the second-floor balcony, entered my room, and found a scene she imagined came right out of a Somerset Maugham story set in Southeast Asia. A lovely little party was underway. The airy and spacious room, measuring about twenty-five by fourteen feet, easily accommodated the multitude of visitors who came to see me. Gathered around my bed and in other places throughout the large room were colleagues (a mixture of British and Americans) from the university where I taught as well as a number of Thai friends laden with fruit and other assorted local goodies. A Japanese friend treated the visitors to a host of delicacies from her restaurant.

Retta walked in and was swept up into the relaxing evening in the hospital room—far from the morbid death scene she had envisioned. No one was uptight. Only the seriousness of my condition marred an otherwise pleasant time. Noui had brought clean sheets and towels and stocked the refrigerator with food. He casually told Ret that Thai tradition dictated that she stay in the room with me. He had been staying, but now it was right for *pee sow,* or older sister, to perform this duty.

o

Retta is by my bedside when they come to take me to the building that houses the suite of operating rooms at Chulalongkorn Hospital. I slip off my gold chain and say, "Please have this; it's not much, but it is the only material thing I have left. Give the Buddha image called *phra uum baat* to Jay, since it is the Buddha for those who are born on Wednesday. We were both born on Wednesdays."

The orderlies and nurses slide me off the bed and onto the stretcher for the trip to the operating room. We go out into a beautiful Thai morning. The sun shines brightly in the clear blue sky overhead. The fresh air and the lush green of the courtyard sweep over me and both comfort and sadden me. I want to stay in nature forever. I ask myself foolishly, *Why can't I enjoy this forever?* Just as quickly I try to center myself. I must not miss the joy and magic of this moment by trying to hold on. I feel my center slip away when I hear myself asking, *Will I feel the joy of morning and the birth of new day, a new season, ever again?*

We move along the balcony, down the elevator, through a covered walkway, across the street to the Operating Room amphitheater. Retta is by my side as we enter the building, turn to the right, and stop at big double doors. She can go no farther. I smile. Say goodbye.

As I am wheeled into the large operating room, I look off to the left and there, squatting and scrubbed, are a group of residents and interns. Nurses scurry about. I see Dr. Chanvit, a face I recognize. I feel better. "*Sawat dee Kuhn maw krap.* Good morning, Doctor," are my last words before I see a nurse approaching me with a mask. Once again a question—*Will this mask be the last thing I ever see?*—forms in my mind. I hear more Thai words, "*tham sabai.* Relax." The nurse puts the mask gently over my mouth and nose. She tells me to breathe gently. It's like following my breath during meditation. I am asleep.

o

I woke up on life-support, momentarily fearful because I hadn't been told that I would be on life-support after the operation. The ventilator scared me, but Retta and the others at my bedside assured me that the life-support was routine after long surgery. I looked down to find that my strings had survived the surgery as well.

I was surprised how quickly I got off the respirator. In twenty-four hours, I was moved back to the pleasant surroundings of my room. I thought my problems were over and all I needed to do was rest, eat, and regain my strength. I progressed amazingly well, and the immediate post-operative period progressed almost routinely. My improvement reassured Retta, and one week later she left for the United States. I promised to take care of myself, and Noui assured Retta that he would watch over me. I told her I wouldn't be able to teach until after the first of the year. I guaranteed her that I would be working out and jogging again by February.

On November 26, eighteen days following the operation, I left Chulalongkorn Hospital to continue my recovery at home. After two days in the small apartment, I ventured into the routine of the world beyond my apartment. Suddenly I found myself outside with cars whizzing by me in the madness of Sukhumvit Road, a major Bangkok street. Panic-stricken, I asked myself, *Where am I? How did I get here? What are all these people doing?* I screamed internally, *Help! Help!*

My confusion, probably a side-effect of the portacaval shunt, resulted in great terror. I have never known such fright. I have been lost at night in the middle of Damascus, not knowing how to get back to camp; wandered outside of Amman with a group of Arabs in a no-man's zone; climbed up thousand-foot boulders; rappelled off steep mountains; navigated whitewater rapids in Canada; driven sports cars at breakneck speeds—in short, done some rather scary things in my life. Nothing compared with suddenly finding myself somewhere and not knowing how I got there. It was like waking up in the midst of a nightmare, but the nightmare went on.

Nightmarish experiences plagued me for the next several days. I was scared to leave my room because I couldn't find my way home. Later, I faced a more fundamental problem. I could not figure out the proper order in which to put on my clothes. Noui found me wandering outside on the main street in my bathing suit. The portacaval shunt had saved my life and stopped the threat of internal bleeding. Had it created this confusion? Would I get better?*

Figuring out daily life confused me. I heard a noise in my apartment and after a time realized it was the phone. I answered and heard, "Hi, John. How are you doing?" At first, the voice in the telephone confused me. I didn't know who was calling me. Then I realized it was my sister, calling from Virginia.

I replied tentatively, "Oh, I'm okay, but a little weak. I'm having problems sleeping and remembering things, but I'm going to make it. Ret, I don't know if I can ever teach again, but I've been thinking maybe I can just run a small hardware store somewhere. There's always a need for an honest person." This conversation, which made absolutely no sense to Retta or any of my family, seemed perfectly logical to me. No one was quite able to understand why I wanted to work in a hardware store. Neither was I.

As I hung up the telephone, trying to make sense of the international phone call from Retta, my friend Allen Lundberg, who lived in the same apartment complex, strolled down to see me. Apparently stunned by what he saw, he exclaimed, "John you've got to go home. You need someone to take care of you." I had known Allen for several years. He is one of those delightful Westerners one often meets in Asia. He had spent years alternating between Bangkok, Kathmandu, and his Los Angeles home. He sold training films. Before that he had been in the Peace Corps in Nepal. Now he—like me—was trying to start a business in Thailand.

"I can't Allen," I resisted. "What would I do? And besides, the bottom line is, I don't have any money at all. It's all gone now. Remember I haven't really worked regularly since May of '83. I don't have any medical insurance in the United States, but the Thai govern-

---

* One of the essential jobs of the liver is storing and releasing important nutrients into the bloodstream. So, in effect, a portion of my blood was both "unclean," in the sense of not being fully cleared of toxins, and nutrient poor. This combination of "unclean" and nutrient-deprived blood affected both my physical endurance and mental capacities. It is much the same thing that can happen to a marathon runner when he uses up his accumulated stores of glycogen and "hits the wall" after several hours of running. While Dr. Sommai warned me about the post-operative complications of shunt surgery, I never fully understood the dangers involved in the operation.

ment hospital and Dr. Sommai will take care of me. I can go upcountry, live in the monastery, and perhaps hold on a little longer."

Lying in bed in the confusion of the sultry Bangkok night, I felt my resistance to Allen's suggestion weaken. I took stock of my options: *I thought after the operation I would be slowed down, but believed, nevertheless, that I could live upcountry or go to the wat. Now I can't do that. I can hardly dress myself. I can't shave. I don't know the TV from the telephone, and everything terrifies me. I can't take care of myself, and it's too much of a burden to place on Noui.*

I concluded: *I'm not going to live long, so now the question is where to die? I can go to Suan Mok* [where I had spent my three years as a Buddhist monk] *and the monks will take care of me until I die, but perhaps that is not fair to Retta. She worries so. Maybe I should die in Virginia. If I can gamble that it won't be costly to die in America, maybe I should go home and die in Fredericksburg.*

Allen brought my breakfast in the morning. I told him, "Perhaps you are right. I should go to America and live with Ret."

"I think that's probably the right thing to do, John."

"But, Allen, there are forms, tax clearances, immigration control, plane reservations, closing up my business, and a million things. I just can't do it now."

"I'll take care of everything," Allen promised.

Getting me ready to return to America was, however, not an easy task. First came financial problems. Allen asked "Where is the money you said you had?"

"Gosh, isn't it in the bank?"

"No."

"Oh, I know I have some money, but I can't remember where I put it. I think Khun Pisarn and Khun Chalong [Thai friends from the Ministry of Interior, where I had a consulting contract] sent 10,000 baht [Thai currency equivalent to approximately $400 at 1987 exchange rates] to the hospital. I'm sure I have it. Ask Noui."

"He hasn't seen it, John."

A day later, Allen found the money tucked away under my futon.

From this point, Allen took over my life. He made calls to Retta almost every other day. He found an easy flight that required only one airline change before depositing me at Dulles Airport in Washington. He contacted my friends in the Interior Ministry to smooth my exit from the country. He bought me a suitcase and instructed me to prepare my clothes for packing.

Finally, everything was set. All I had to do was go with him to pick up my airline ticket and sign the credit card form. Just doing this fairly simple task of everyday life—signing a credit slip—would prove to be an awesome task, I feared. "Allen, I can't sign my name. My hand shakes too much since the operation"*

"John, you've got two days. Practice and practice."

"Noui," Allen instructed, "make John practice signing his name every day."

I felt like a fresh-air kid being sent to summer camp when Allen came in a Thai International limousine to pick me up on the morning of December 15, 1985, for my flight to Hong Kong, Seattle, and Washington, D.C. I was given instructions, shown my ticket several times. Then Allen gave me my spending money for the trip home. He had changed baht, the Thai currency, into dollars and he explained to me all about my money. He gave me a letter for Retta and letters from my doctors to show the airline. At least I was spared the indignity of the big sign around my neck with my name and address.

We left the apartment. It was another beautiful morning with a bright sky. I promised the delegation of friends there to see me off, "I'll be right back, just like last time. Trust me." I lied. I knew I was never coming back. I just couldn't say it to myself or anyone else. I couldn't cry. I couldn't laugh. Everything was swirling outside me, yet I felt empty and alone inside. I have never felt so alone in my entire life. I don't even remember saying goodbye. It seems like I went from my apartment to the airplane with nothing in between. I looked out the window and saw the green rice paddies of my beloved Thailand slipping into a giant Manet canvas of green. I was headed to a place called "home," for a special rendezvous with my karma, my deeds.

---

* As I later learned, this was a side-effect both of the operation and of a poorly functioning liver. The condition, known as encephalopathy, is a kind of degenerative brain disease. In my case, it most likely was the result of toxins and lack of nutrients in the blood because of the damaged liver.

2

Welcome Home

*. . . if in order to live it is necessary not to live, then
what's it all for?*
Solzhenitsyn, *The Gulag Archipelago*

Liver disease destroys you physically, mentally, and emotionally.
Never-ending fatigue and subtle changes in mental functioning
break down your will and undermine your confidence. This in turn
places special strains on friends and family. My decline not only
frustrated me, but also exacted a special burden on those around me. I
was living with Retta, who had to learn to treat me like a child without,
at the same time, making me feel patronized. Every encounter required
patience and a deft sense of balance. Retta and I learned this almost
every day, as even the most routine task became as complex as
navigating an elaborate maze.

Television offered a confusing set of controls that appeared as
complex to me as those of a spacecraft. "Retta, I can't seem to turn on
the television. How do you do it?" I had phoned and interrupted her in
the middle of her teaching art classes at Stafford High School.

"John, first, you have to find the button and turn it on."

"I can't find the button."

"Do you see the box on the set? That box has a series—in a row,
next to each other—of buttons and it's the last button on the right. It says
'power.' That turns on the TV."

"Oh, okay. Wait let me see if I can do that. . . . Good! I did it, but
how do I get the different channels?"

Other simple tasks of life around the house proved equally as challenging. One day, I turned on the water and couldn't figure out how to turn it off. Once again Retta got a panic call at school. She calmed me down and carefully explained how to turn the faucet off. Her days were filled with adolescent prattle at high school and calming a brother at home who was frequently scared by living a life severely handicapped due to liver disease.

In the midst of my struggle to master the baffling routine of daily life, Jay, Ret, and I decided that I must try to qualify for medical assistance. On a cold, grey December day, Retta bundled me in her MGB and drove me to the Social Security office. It is difficult to describe your feelings when you are forced to slink into some office filled with strangers and say you can't take care of yourself. I felt I had reached the end and noted in my diary, "Am now at the bottom." I learned all about Social Security, S.S.I., Medicaid, and Food Stamps in a sequential process that began at the local Social Security office with an interview and a multitude of forms, continued with reviews at Regional Offices, examinations by a physician and psychologist, and finally concluded at the welfare office.

I was grateful that the government apparently designed the system for someone with a third-grade comprehension level. Officials explained everything carefully, repeating instructions and questions many times. The simplicity was necessary. I couldn't follow a more involved conversation. Often Retta had to answer for me. At every stage people dealt with me kindly, thoughtfully, and respectfully. Although the forms didn't seem designed for my situation—"How much did you have to lift in your last job? What was your average hourly wage?"—the system responded, although at times slowly and awkwardly.

There were other anomalies that startled some of the participants in the routine. I went to a doctor for a physical to certify that I was handicapped. After the examination, the doctor puzzled, "I will certify you handicapped, but you know I've never examined a Ph.D. for this status before. Most of the people I examine for Social Security disability haven't even graduated from elementary school."

I guess he was trying to make me feel better.

What is the sound of one hand clapping?

Zen koan

It's April 11, 1986, a beautiful Virginia spring afternoon, my day of reckoning. I am heading for an appointment with Dr. David Rice at the Pratt Clinic in Fredericksburg to get a definite answer, in plain English, about my future. I know the final word looms ever closer. All around me spring celebrates rebirth and new life. The flowers are in full color. The Bradford pear trees float everywhere like great puffs of white against the blue sky. Other trees are filling up green. Virginia's famed dogwood is in bloom. Birth, newness, freshness, and hope surround me while I face winter. My life is entering its final season. I can no longer care for myself or live alone.

I am scared. I am fearful of American doctors. I regard them as businessmen. The irony of my situation strikes me. Dr. Sommai, I recall to myself, took Jay's charge very seriously and committed himself and his institution to my care. In a Third World country, care came first and money second. In the United States, I know money comes first. My thoughts wander. *I don't know what to expect. Gosh, I was forty-five before I ever entered an emergency room in the United States, when Charlie McAdams stitched me up after a running accident. Charlie's an American doctor, but he's a friend. I don't even know Dr. Rice.*

I enter the office. The receptionist asks me to fill out a two-page form that contains seemingly endless questions. Retta's not here to help me like she was the day at Social Security. After I struggle through the forms, the nurse ushers me into one of Dr. Rice's small examining areas. He enters the room with a sheaf of papers, obviously the results of lab tests I took last week. He looks like a doctor; he's calm and quiet. The situation is awkward for both of us. Small talk and then, "John, given what I see now, and in light of your past medical history, you can probably hang on for six months to a year."

"What does 'hang on' mean, doctor? 'Live?' "

"Yes."

"Is there any cure?"

"No."

At that moment, my life assumes an intensity beyond anything I have ever experienced—an intensity that creates a strange kind of euphoria. It makes a drug experience or a meditative trance seem mild by comparison. No anger, no denial, no bargaining, nothing . . . but everything. A sudden stream of unconnected, disjointed thoughts, like a James Joyce stream-of-consciousness novel, flowed quickly through my mind.

wow what is this feeling it's the most intense trip i've ever had but i'm not on a thing no lights no sounds no warmth nothing but a very strange feeling the snow is purple as it falls on the country club look at that painting yes the one that looks like the air conditioner filter see it in three d yes of course i am a crow and the leaf is falling up look at the wine fly through the air and it splashes drop by drop off gary's face and randy if you lean forward you'll fall right to the floor ah ohm to my childrens children can see it oh the sounds of the ocean are beautiful and look how i can stop the rain and see each drop hit the leaves of the trees in the jungle i am breathing in and breathing out now slower now longer and even longer and longer i may even stop breathing altogether centering i am focused at the tip of my nose and i am slowly settling into jhana i am warm ah i like it but now it will all go away how long have i been like this what does the doctor think i can't hear him and i can barely see him i am not sure i can move speak or see i don't feel bad i don't feel good i don't feel i'm not scared i'm not reassured i'm not empty but i'm not full i'm not angry i don't feel denial i don't feel acceptance do i feel anything i feel everything and nothing mai pen rai yes truly mai pen rai it doesn't matter nothing matters yet everything matters thank you mai pen rai don't sweat it ah don't you see it now it's the sound of one hand clapping yes now i understand mai pen rai is the real heart of chun nun eng, the very way of being but wait i've already said this when the university students used to visit the monastery for meditation and dhamma talks oh but now i really understand it i was so glib before let me have my old words back i understand now but don't have better words oh what difference does it make anyway mai pen rai

"Thank you doctor."
I walk home. It is still a pretty spring day. Nothing's happened.

O

Death. I knew I had few doubts about death. I reconciled myself to it a long time ago, but not until Dr. Rice's words did I begin waiting for death. His words changed nothing. Only one thing really seemed to bother me: I would be forced to undertake the next step on the path without money. It's tough to have to figure out the end of your life and face death, but, in addition, to worry about finances—particularly whether family and friends should have to make a major expenditure that may alter their lives—is a needless complication.

On May 1, 1986, following Dr. Rice's advice to see a specialist in liver disease at the Medical College of Virginia, Jay and I traveled to Richmond. I knew that a liver transplant might be discussed, but even before meeting the new doctor, I understood I did not have a strong case for transplant because transplants generally had not been successful on hepatitis B patients. Also, I knew that previous liver surgery, like my operation last year in Bangkok, considerably complicated the prospects of transplant. Nevertheless, I had no feeling of desperately clinging to a long-shot chance of preserving my life. In fact, I was not exactly sure what was in my mind as Jay and I drove the fifty miles south down Interstate 95 to Richmond. I just seemed to be doing what came to me at the moment and did not worry about anything else. I was merely taking the next step in a series of events leading from my first getting sick in Bangkok almost three years ago.

I realized that I was calm because I thought, *After all what worse news can I receive than I have already heard from Dr. Rice?* I went through my usual anxiety of meeting yet another new doctor—especially one in an impersonal American academic setting who headed the liver transplant program at the Medical College of Virginia. However, my fear evaporated almost as soon as I entered his office. He was a very busy man, but as soon as his door closed, I felt that he shut out the world and that nothing else mattered but me, his patient.

He moved quickly to involve me in my future. I understood almost at once that he would never tell me what to do. Time slid by quickly and easily. He never looked at his watch nor talked on the phone. He looked me squarely in the eye. We talked for over an hour. I felt comfortable and knew I had stumbled into a relationship with an extraordinary man—Robert L. Carithers, Jr., M.D.

We talked about my medical history, my illness in Thailand, my life and values. He spoke to me without a hint of judgment in his voice. My life of wandering did not seem strange to him. We used this first hour getting to know each other, and didn't get down to the intricacies of medical diagnosis and transplant because he wanted to see the results of blood tests and other examinations at MCV before we decided on a course to pursue. Perhaps some treatment short of transplant could help with my condition. Or, on the other hand, there might be factors that would totally rule out transplant. Only time and further analysis would answer that question. He seemed mainly concerned to learn something about me and how I viewed my life.

"John, what do you feel about the quality of your life now?"

"It's terrible, Dr. Carithers. I can't do anything for myself. I can't live by myself, and I am slowly getting more dependent on others. It is no life at all."

"You know, John, the only reason I am in this field of medicine is that a successful liver transplant can restore a high quality of life. The aim of our program is to enable you to lead a high-quality, independent life. We do not want to create semi-invalids, but rather people who are fully functional. If we can't do that, the program makes no sense."

This reassured me, because I feared initially that the medical faculty was just another branch of the university in which research came first and patients second. I knew that the "prestige order" in medical universities held the researcher in higher regard than the clinician. I understood that because I knew from my own experience that the university administrations valued a publisher more highly than a teacher. Carithers appeared to me to be a fresh and humane voice inside the walls of academe and medicine. Nevertheless, my academic background forced me to ask, "Where did you go to school?"

"My undergraduate degree is from the University of North Carolina, and my medical degree from University of Pennsylvania. I returned to Chapel Hill for my internship and residency."

He'd said the right words. "I love Chapel Hill. You know I taught in the U.N.C. system at Charlotte and spent much time at Chapel Hill. Did you know James Taylor's father, who was Dean of the Medical School? I think if I were to live any place in the United States it would be Chapel Hill—as long as Dean Smith is coach of the 'Heels."

Carithers, too, is a basketball fan and we recounted our own personal favorite Tarheel players and games, reserving our most lavish praise for Michael Jordan and the 1982 championship game. For Carolina fans, it is a necessary bonding to recall where you were for that great game.

"Of course," I continued, "you probably would not have taken courses with any of my friends on the faculty, because you were one of those science people and stayed in the labs."

"On the contrary," he corrected me, "I was an English major." Responding to my stunned look, he added, "I have always had this fairly strong feeling about being well-rounded. It accounts for my motivation towards sports. I lost my academic scholarship by devoting too much time trying to make the Carolina baseball team. This same motivation made me want to follow an academic course different from that of other pre-meds. Luckily my advisor at U.N.C. was an Associate Dean for Student Affairs, who supported my desire to major in English as a pre-med."

"Who are your favorites?" I ask excitedly, never having expected to have a literary discussion with a doctor.

"Faulkner, Hemingway, and Steinbeck. Of course, I loved the macho stuff in Hemingway. Steinbeck's sense of the downtrodden, particularly in *The Grapes of Wrath*, and his social stuff always appealed to me. You know, there's enough socialist in me to believe every person has a right to medical care. But, of course, my great love was Faulkner."

"That's fantastic," I continued. "My Ph.D. was in Southern political history. What about Faulkner did you like?"

"Because of my grandfather's Mississippi background, I got very interested in V.K. Ratliff, the sewing-machine salesman character in *The Hamlet, The Town and The Mansion.* I liked Faulkner because he was different—no one was reading him for pleasure then. I even did an honors course and senior thesis on Faulkner. My advisor was Harry Russell, a marvelous old man."

"I think I am going to like this doctor," I told Jay as we left and returned to Fredericksburg.

Joan took me back to MCV two weeks later for my second appointment with the Nutrition Center of the hospital. First, I had to see the dietician, who put me on a regime of 30 grams of protein a day. This restriction changed my whole diet, because just two pieces of toast, butter, and cereal and milk and juice for breakfast almost exceeded my daily allotment of protein. Ever since the portacaval shunt, I had followed a vegetarian diet. Now my food was even more strictly controlled, because even many of my vegetarian items were high in protein. I needed food for strength, but too much protein, because it is metabolized in the liver, could send me into coma and death. It was another of the seemingly endless Catch 22s of my life.

In the afternoon, I walked into Dr. Carithers' office for the final word on my condition. He confirmed Dr. Rice's judgment. He got right to the point. "John, a transplant is your only hope. Without it your life expectancy is maybe a year, six months, maybe less. One of the most difficult tasks of liver transplants is timing. It's a risky operation and we don't want to take any time away from you that you might normally have by subjecting you to an operation that may end your life. But rest assured, your life is almost over without a transplant."

He never said "you must have a transplant." Rather, he encouraged me to make the decision. "John, I must be frank with you. You have two enormous obstacles to overcome. First, Dr. Thomas Starzl, who originated the operation, never was successful with a patient who has had a portacaval shunt. And second, you have no money. MCV is not like the more strict transplant centers, and we will make every effort to work with you as a citizen of the Commonwealth if you can come up with about twenty-five percent of the costs up front, as a down payment."

(Carithers hated to talk finances with a patient, but he had no choice in my case. Before giving its permission to re-start the liver transplant program in 1984, the hospital administration, fearing that liver transplants might bankrupt the hospital, made the doctors promise to undertake a financial screening of potential transplant patients. My situation forced Carithers to keep his promise.)

"But, Dr. Carithers," I protested, "I've qualified for Medicaid, and that certainly should be enough for the down payment."

"Yes," he responded grimly, "but Virginia Medicaid, unlike almost every other state, does not pay for liver transplants. It is so silly that it will pay for hospitalization for the transplant evaluation and for immunosuppressive drugs after the transplant, but not for the transplant itself."

I returned to Fredericksburg with the possibility of transplant looming in my mind, but I was just getting used to the idea when, suddenly, my life almost ended before the process could begin.

On a Friday night in May, I felt very weak and by Saturday morning I was running a high fever. I had some type of infection, which is always a threat to people with liver disease. Joan located Dr. Rice on his day off, and he agreed to meet me in his office. It was our first meeting since our fateful encounter in April.

He looked worried and put me in the hospital. An array of doctors paraded through my room to examine me. I heard a group of them in consultation with Jay in the hall outside my room. For a while there was talk of airlifting me to Richmond, but since no one could locate Dr. Carithers, the doctors in Fredericksburg were afraid that I might get overlooked in the big, impersonal medical center in Richmond. Dr. Rice felt that he could treat me in Fredericksburg over the weekend.

Jay called Retta, who was in Baltimore visiting friends, and she rushed back to Fredericksburg. I figured Jay had told her that death was eminent, and that's why she returned. But I survived the life-threatening hours, responded to medication, and left Fredericksburg's Mary Washington Hospital after a ten-day stay. This brought my total to ninety-five days in hospitals in nine separate trips since my first stay in St. Louis Hospital in Bangkok in February 1984. I wondered if I would live long enough for a transplant. I had read that a sizeable portion of people needing transplants die while they are on the waiting list. I wasn't even on the list yet.

Three days after my discharge from Mary Washington, Jay and I were in Dr. Carithers' office again. "What do you know about liver transplants?" he asked us.

"Not much."

Carithers then explained briefly. "Dr. Starzl did the first transplant in Colorado in 1965, and the first successful transplant in 1968. No one was very enthusiastic about liver transplants because the best survival rate that Starzl was ever able to achieve was between thirty and forty percent. Because of the expense involved and the relatively low rate of success, many felt it was not worth getting into.

"At that time, MCV already had a well-established kidney and heart transplant program, and in 1968, Dr. Hume, Dr. Lee, and MCV surgeons began performing liver transplants. By 1969, they had done four, and one patient lived a year and a half. At that time, the consensus of the surgeons around the country was that it wasn't a feasible operation. In 1980, Starzl moved to Pittsburgh and was able to get cyclosporine [the pioneering drug to control rejection of transplanted organs] and with that, the success rate started climbing. In the mid-1980s, MCV re-started its liver transplant program. This year we plan to do around twenty-five, and we hope eventually to be doing fifty a year. If you are accepted, you would be among our first thirty patients.

"You must both understand, though, that your case, John, is special because of the portacaval shunt. Our surgeon, Dr. Mendez, may be willing to do the operation, but he wants to be sure that both of you and the others in your family understand the enormous risks and odds involved. Normally in our program the pre-transplant and post-transplant care and evaluation are done by the medical department, and the surgeon is involved only in the final technical details of acceptance. He, of course, has the final word in determining who we transplant. But normally he is not involved too heavily in the evaluation process. This case is different. He wants to see John and the family before committing finally to the operation. He wants to satisfy himself that you all understand the risk."

"John doesn't really have much of a choice, does he?" Jay asked.

"People always have a choice," Dr. Carithers replied quietly. That mild statement illustrated his frank way of dealing with patients. Patients, he believes, must be directly involved in decisions about their care. They are not children or inferiors to be dictated to. (Several years earlier, he explained to us, his church had asked him to organize a program involving ethical choices in medicine. He arranged the program and explained the scientific and medical issues involved. He admired the lay person's ability to grasp the issues, deal with them, and reach a sound moral and medical conclusion. "This experience," he explained, "changed my practice of medicine forever.")

My time to decide had come. Carithers looked squarely at me. "John, I haven't heard you say yet that you really want a transplant."

"The risk doesn't bother me, but the money is a concern. It is difficult for me to ask people to give money for what is such a long-shot chance. I can fight the system, but I am not sure I can engage in fundraising. Ray Wallace, one of my best friends from college days, who now lives in Richmond, has promised to conduct a quiet drive among my college classmates. You must understand, however, that I have lived all over the world, and therefore do not have a core of people in any one place to call upon. Getting the system changed would be much easier."

"What are we talking about in the realm of cost?" Jay asked. "My colleagues in Pittsburgh tell me that $150,000 is the minimum for such an operation."

"As a public institution, we are committed to helping the people of the Commonwealth," Carithers replied, "and we do not have to be as strict as a private university hospital. The hospital has agreed that we can put you on the list if we have approximately a quarter of the estimated cost, around $20,000, as a down payment, and a commitment in good faith to try to pay the balance."

Jay replied quietly, "Well, for the first time since I learned of John's varices, I'm encouraged. There may be some real hope. What's our next step?"

Carithers looked at me. "You must enter MCV for a week-long medical evaluation for a transplant very soon."

"How soon?"

"As soon as possible."

3

MCV

A man of knowledge lives by acting not by thinking about
acting; nor by thinking about what he will think about
after he has acted; a man of knowledge divines a path
with heart and follows it.
Don Juan, *A Separate Reality*

My future hung in the balance during an intensive pre-transplant evaluation that followed. An eerie feeling gently engulfed me in this situation. The tension was so unusual—a tenseness that in a strange way was not at all unsettling. Previous tests confirmed that I was going to die. Now I had to await the results of still more tests to see if I was going to be offered a chance, albeit small, to continue the fight. "Don't think so much—just be attentively aware," my meditation teachers often told me as I learned to calm my mind. This time I took their advice and went through my life-or-death evaluation like a spectator playing a role on a large stage.

My stage was the Medical College of Virginia in Richmond (the medical branch of Virginia Commonwealth University). MCV's place in the city's emerging skyline had been overshadowed recently by the maze of new construction that has transformed the downtown Richmond landscape. For years, its imposing red brick tower dominated the skyscape of the city in the same manner that the smell of cigarette factories in the nearby bottoms by the James River dominated the nostrils of visitors to this centuries-old capital of Virginia, also the former home to the Confederate government.

41

MCV today stands in an area that witnessed momentous events of American history. On Church Hill, just across the James River from the hospital, is St. John's Church, where Patrick Henry delivered his "Give me liberty or give me death" oration on the eve of the American Revolution. Across Broad Street from MCV is the Greek revival Virginia state capitol building designed by Thomas Jefferson. Also in close proximity and now virtually dwarfed by the new MCV tower is Jefferson Davis's home, the White House of the Confederacy, which represents yet another part of the city's long history.

Both my father and brother had graduated from MCV, and I knew its history well. For many years MCV mirrored Virginia. It was a sleepy medical college, mainly training small-town physicians to deliver care to the people of the state. It shared with most other state medical schools in the South a local and provincial mission in common with the outlook of the region. Private schools—Duke in North Carolina, Emory in Georgia, Vanderbilt in Tennessee, and, of course, Johns Hopkins in Maryland—dominated medicine in the South. In recent years, MCV had climbed into the ranks of nationally recognized medical universities.

Transplantation brought its first international acclaim. The school's clinical transplant program began experimentally in 1957, when Dr. David Hume, who had recently come to MCV from Boston, performed a kidney transplant between twins. Transplantation remained an experimental therapy until 1962, when it became an official part of the medical program. By 1986, it had become the longest-lived program of its kind in the United States. By the time I arrived, MCV's surgeons had already performed over 700 kidney transplants.

In 1966, Christiaan Barnard traveled to Richmond to study transplantation techniques with Dr. Hume and Dr. H.M. Lee, the current head of the clinical transplant program. In 1968, another early MCV pioneer, Dr. Richard Lower, performed the hospital's first heart transplant. In fact, MCV and Stanford University claim the two longest continuous heart transplant programs in the country. The history of the college reassured me. I never considered going anywhere else.

I began the evaluation on a Monday morning, knowing that by Friday I would learn whether the doctors planned to give me a chance to live a little longer. I settled into the routine at MCV quickly and easily. After all, hospitals had become almost a second home since February 1984, when my life began centering on doctors and medical processes. Everything appeared well-organized, and I felt secure. I repeated my medical and personal history dozens of times to an assortment of interns, residents, and medical students, never failing to elicit strange looks from the assorted chroniclers. I learned the routine quickly and began answering questions even before they were asked.

I felt like I was in a scene from *The Right Stuff,* preparing for a space mission. The team hauled me from one end of the hospital complex (spread over three downtown blocks) to another for a variety of exotic tests by an array of well-trained technicians operating a battery of expensive, high-tech equipment that appeared to come right out of science fiction. Only it wasn't a story! It was real and happening to me. It just seemed other-worldly.

Apparently in order to save me, the doctors first had to reduce me to some kind of machine and calibrate me. I quickly learned that the person, the human being, is easily lost in the technological tangle of modern medicine. A kind of strange uneasiness settled over me as the evaluation process unfolded. I was not apprehensive about life and death, but rather about what might happen to my spirituality in this whole process. The process itself—not the thought of receiving another person's organ or the continual discomfort of the struggle—is what gave me the most concern. This worry remained, for me, the most unsettling of all the traumas of my illness.

Here, during evaluation, I really began my contest with the medical profession for control of my life. It was to be my most difficult struggle. A common theme in stories about the legal profession is that lawyers often lose sight of their clients in an overzealous attempt to "win." It is less well known, but equally true of the medical profession, that many doctors lose sight of patients' spiritual well-being in an equally passionate attempt to "win." American doctors in particular seem defeated by death.

I was scanned, injected, and inspected. First came the scans and tests: spleen scans, abdomen scans, blood scans, pulmonary scans, scans of scans, and then so many blood tests and biopsies that I felt I would need a transfusion to replace all the blood drawn for tests. The team assigned a young intern to make immune system tests, so I had a series of interesting little scrapes covered by patches on several places up and down my arms.

Next came the soundings: ultrasounds, the echocardiograms and hepatic arterograms, EEGs and EKGs—I felt like I was in a New Deal relief program with all the initials and acronyms I kept hearing. The machines terrified me.

On his first visit, I elicited a promise from Dr. Carithers not to make extraordinary efforts to keep me alive. I knew that sounded funny, because remarkable measures had already been taken to keep me alive to this point. What I meant was that I didn't wish to "live" as little more than a vegetable, maintained by machines and feeding tubes. He explained the living will and the Virginia Natural Death Act, and I determined to execute the necessary papers as soon as I left the hospital.

Through it all, the staff at MCV remained patient and caring. The technicians and doctors took time to explain every machine and let me look at the scopes that showed my liver and other internal organs. The staff always spoke to me in nontechnical terms, avoiding medical double-talk. I was enormously relieved, since I had heard horror stories of the impersonality of major medical research facilities and of state-run hospitals.

During my evaluation, I got to know more members of the transplant team. First was Ann Reid Priest, a critical-care nurse specialist, who coordinated the program and was the major link with the patients. She is an extraordinary woman and uniquely qualified to bring a personal element that balanced the technology of modern medicine. As a woman, she brought the special qualities of her gender to the art of healing. She nurtures and cares for people and understands that medicine is more than machines, diagnosis, and prescription. She's done all the traditional masculine things as well: a Master of Science degree in nursing from the University of Virginia, where she won the Louise Mellon Fellowship and received an award for outstanding research for her thesis, "The Moral Reasoning Process of Critical Care Nurses." She also followed the correct path in academic nursing, with publications, seminars, and workshops.

Ann is a team player and by temperament does not think in terms of win or lose, but rather of resolving issues and keeping everyone working together, a feminine characteristic often downplayed in a male-dominated profession. As a result she was philosophically predisposed to hear my observations about Asian medicine. I told her about my experiences in a system that, in many ways, was not win- and male-dominated, but rather was more devoted to care.

Ann explained what would happen during the transplant process and said I would spend more time with nurses than with physicians, because nurses, "by virtue of their training, treat the range of human response to illness, while physicians by virtue of their training only diagnose and treat illness." Ann comforted me amidst the labyrinth of impersonal machines.

o

"I don't like psychologists," I told the transplant team's psychologist, Mary Ellen Olbrisch, when she entered my room. "But since this is part of the evaluation, I suppose we had better get on with it." We were certainly not off to a promising beginning.

I explained my problem with psychologists to her. "I just don't believe you can talk anyone into mental health, and besides, I have bad memories of psychologists. My first wife—well, actually, I've only had one—was a psychologist and I have taken all your silly tests, which are articulations of the obvious."

Mary Ellen and I talked for over forty-five minutes. We discussed my personal history and my spiritual life. I told her that cost was my major fear of the transplant and that I did not want to be a burden to my family. We talked about her Texas background (training in Austin) and about her spirituality, which was rooted in the Roman Catholic Church. To me, Mary Ellen seemed caught between the nurturing characteristics of women, her Roman Catholic religious faith, and the cold detachment of the aloof social scientist. As with Ann Reid and Bob Carithers, the church is an important part of her life.

I found the experience not nearly as bad as I had anticipated. I liked her, but didn't expect to see her again. I felt that I could probably handle the psychological and philosophical issues of transplant surgery and recovery on my own, based on the years I had already spent in philosophical search and meditation.

Mary Ellen recorded her conclusions of our initial interview in the records for the transplant team's final evaluation: "He is an extroverted, serene individual, his judgment is good and is coping well with current situation; however, he is concerned about extreme measures to prolong life. He may also tend to be impatient about some of the unpredictability of hospital care. He is an excellent candidate for liver transplant from a psychological perspective, but due to financial concerns and wishes not to be indebted to family, patient may reject surgery option."

○

"You're a Buddhist, aren't you?" A lovely Asian nurse startled me while waking me in the middle of the night.

"Yes, how did you know," I asked, stunned by the question.

"By the strings on your wrists," she replied, referring to the *sai sila* that Noui had tied around my wrists at Chulalongkorn Hospital in Bangkok eight months ago. "I, too, am a Buddhist and I understand the symbolism and importance of the strings. I sometimes feel great confusion between the East and the West. You're here for a transplant evaluation, aren't you?"

"Yes," I answered, opening a long conversation about karma, *mai pen rai, chun nun eng,* and the elements of Eastern and Western philosophy. She left after about fifteen or twenty minutes.

The Asian nurse wrote in my record, "He talks freely about his Buddhist beliefs. Believes in karma—not morose, matter of factly speaks of continued life or death, that all is cyclic and predetermined. He told me he would like to live longer if possible, but if not, that would be fate and not for him to decide."

○

"Hello, Mr. Robbins, I'm Rick Liverman, the social worker on the transplant team." I looked up and saw a bright, cheerful, earnest, dark-haired young man in his twenties. I thought to myself as I tried to be pleasant to Rick, *Is this never going to end? First the psychologists, now the social worker. Are they going to bring in Jerry Falwell next?*

"Why do I need to see a social worker?" I wondered in a less than cordial opener. Rick never quite answered my question, but somehow he became a significant part of my experience at MCV. I'm not really sure what he did. He met with my friends during the fundraising. He talked to my sister and sister-in-law. But most of all he seemed to care. He became another human balance to the machines.

o

I was relaxing from a round of tests when suddenly I heard, in a Spanish accent, "Mr. Robbins, I'm Dr. Mendez, the surgeon." I looked up to see the bearded surgical whiz of the liver transplant program making one of his rare pre-op visits to a transplant candidate. He wanted to make sure I understood the risk of the surgery after the portacaval shunt. I was a little wary of a surgeon who wanted to undertake what many regarded a long-shot effort. I knew about research, and I knew the politics of grants and funding for research projects and programs. Why was he willing to take a chance on a case that might spoil his and MCV's statistics? He wanted to know about me. I wanted to know about him.

First, he explained the complications of the portacaval shunt. Previous surgery in the same area of the transplant vastly increases the number of raw surfaces that might bleed. Bleeding is a major problem in liver transplants, and the previous shunt surgery raised the distinct possibility of uncontrolled hemorrhaging that would end my life. In addition, the prior surgery might make it impossible to dissect and separate all the vessels leading to and from the liver, as well as those that anchor it in the body. As a result, once he opened me up, he might find that the operation was simply not feasible. If that happened, I would most likely die on the operating table.

Despite all the sophisticated tests and scans and high-tech machines for charting the internal organs, there was still no way to be positive that the transplant was possible before actually opening up the patient. It was, as he explained, a big gamble. But, he assured me, he was willing to take it. Why was he willing to take the gamble? "I believe that medicine is a duty, a sacred profession in the European tradition. Because my father was a physician, I was brought up with the sense of service and I have never felt that any patient was an imposition. And of course," he continued, "in this type of work, we welcome the opportunity of obtaining a new experience or doing something new—but we take it with trepidation, and that is why I want to be sure you understand how very sick you are and the enormous risk you are taking."

How should I answer him? I thought to myself. I wanted to live, but I didn't want to live in a way that created too many problems for me. I didn't want to beg. I wanted to remain unattached from the struggle for life itself. My answer involved explaining a spiritual view that I had spent a long time trying to understand myself. I tried to maintain the same kind of attitude as I had in my conversation with the Asian nurse two nights before when we talked about karma. I sought to maintain a balance between acceptance and resignation, between enthusiasm and hopelessness.

I asked myself, *How can I make him understand* <u>*uphekkha,*</u> *tranquility? How can I make him understand that I am willing to fight for my life, but I surely will not beg for the chance? Or that I will not attach to the fight? How can I make him understand* <u>*sunnata,*</u> *or emptiness? Or that I want a state of mind that produces no deeds, no action to influence the future?* I was struggling to explain points of Buddhist metaphysics that governed my life when suddenly I knew that words made no difference whatsoever. He would have to understand me by what I did, not by what I said.

"I understand the risk, Dr. Mendez. I am quite willing to take it. I do not want to be kept alive by machines, and I have explained already to Dr. Carithers that I want to be able to live a high-quality life after the surgery."

I had no idea what he thought when he left the room. Perhaps I should have tried to explain with more words. *Mai pen rai*, I repeated to myself. It really doesn't matter anyway.

o

I felt no particular anxiety when Dr. Carithers walked into my hospital room Friday afternoon, the sixth day of June 1986, to tell me the results. I was suddenly very calm. Throughout the week I was never nervous. I was much more on edge waiting for my final oral exams for my Ph.D. I have felt more apprehension waiting for a mechanic's assessment of my car.

"John, we see no reason medically why we can't attempt the transplant. You are a reasonable candidate for a transplant and you have no other option."

I didn't know whether to be thankful or fearful of the surgery. *Mai pen rai*, I repeated to myself. It doesn't matter. Nothing does.

o

"Why did you take this case, Jerry?" H.M. Lee asked Gerardo Mendez-Picon, his colleague in vascular and transplant surgery. The two men presented a classic contrast as they studied the charts in their shabby quarters in the Nelson Clinic, where the MCV staff doctors have their offices. Outwardly they couldn't have been more different. Hyung Mo Lee, a quiet, smooth-skinned, slight, gentlemanly Korean-American came to MCV in 1955 and since 1973 had been the Director of the internationally acclaimed Clinical Transplant program. His manner gave no indication that he was a distinguished physician. He was certainly anything but TV's image of a surgeon. "St. Elsewhere's" Mark Craig he was not. Lee had been at MCV for thirty-two years and his students were well-known surgeons in their own right throughout the nation and the world. In fact, one student, Christiaan Barnard, had performed the world's first human heart transplant. Lee simply did not need to impress; he knew his worth and his ability. His honors and professional memberships fill over a page of his vitae, and his publications run beyond two hundred.

Gerardo Joaquin Angel Mendez-Picon, another case altogether, lived up to TV's image of a surgeon. A Latin version of Mark Craig, he arrived at MCV in 1969 from Spain by way of the University of Kansas Medical Center as a Junior Assistant Resident of Surgery. In 1981, he became an Associate Professor of Surgery and by 1986 was regarded as the program's top liver transplant surgeon. Conjure up a vision of Lee, then think of everything opposite, and you come up with Gerardo Mendez-Picon, *El Padrino*, the Spanish Godfather. Mendez was bearded, stocky, loud, cocky, difficult, a great ego. Everyone knew when Jerry Mendez was around. Flamboyant and colorful, Mendez could be a public relations man's nightmare. Outspoken and opinionated, he was the bright light in liver transplant surgery. Without hesitation, he told everyone within hearing distance, "Liver surgery is where it's at . . . liver transplantation is the most difficult and demanding surgery we do today." Mendez, as people grudgingly admitted, knew what he was talking about. He had come from the ranks of vascular surgery and kidney transplants to liver transplant. He had the best statistics in the country.

Although different in temperament, both doctors agreed on the preeminence of the surgeon in transplantation. Lee was fond of citing the work of MCV's David Hume and other early pioneers in transplantation, who, as surgeons, had recognized and described transplantation not as a separate surgical technical exercise, but as a science. Lee often cited a 1961 article in the *Journal of Clinical Investigation* that he described as a classic of scientific investigation into transplant and that began the history of viewing transplantation as a scientific medical problem. Subsequent research in transplantation was built on this model.

Lee had trained Mendez well. Mendez, with less tact than Lee, asserted that surgeons were first in the transplant field, knew more about the subject, and were, of course, preeminent. Doctors from almost every other speciality—for example, internists—became interested in transplants only after surgeons had become the pioneers in the field. Surgeons are the ballerinas of medicine. Mendez could exasperate his colleagues on the transplant team with his constant assertion, "Surgery always runs transplant. Of course, we may consult, but we are in charge." For that matter, Mendez could exasperate almost anyone, not just members of the transplant team: other nurses and doctors, administrators, secretaries, patients. Nobody, however, questioned his skill or his genuine commitment to the patient. His explosiveness was written off to his Latin background. Ann Reid Priest would say, "We all know that Jerry has to say surgery runs transplant, but that's okay. We know how to placate him."

As the elder, Lee had a special relationship with Mendez. He recalls fondly the day when he interviewed the young Spaniard for his residency appointment. Mendez's cockiness, self-assurance, and, above all, his coolness impressed Lee. Mendez, he notes, told him, "I went to a good school in Spain. My father is a physician. I want to be the best and I think I'm good. If I don't get accepted, I'll try again."

That impressed Lee. "He didn't sweat. He had ego, confidence, and knew what he wanted in the future. In the meantime, he wasn't tense and anxious as hell that you wouldn't take him. Compared to others, he was calmer." Surgeons are a special breed of doctors who look at each other critically and enjoy turning up the pressure. Ultimately what set Mendez apart in Lee's mind was that "he didn't sweat." That's really important in the macho world of surgeons, the marines of medicine.

The two men shared another important experience. They were both foreigners in a program that had a history of hostility to foreigners. In the late fifties, Lee survived Dr. David Hume's purge of foreign residents at MCV. Lee had done his time in the labs to gain the confidence of Dr. Hume, who came to MCV from Boston to ramrod the school's transplant program. Lee participated with him in one of the early, seminal articles on transplantation and, in the sixties, became a trusted member of the team. Perhaps, he told Hume in 1969, it was time to bring in another foreigner. Mendez was Lee's man.

"Why did you take this case, Jerry? Transplant after portacaval shunt is a very deep hole indeed." Lee asked Mendez because the senior surgeon knew that standard surgical thinking dictated that you try to avoid getting into a deep hole. Mendez was not required to ask Lee's permission to do the transplant, but they talked about difficult cases. Lee knew Mendez never shrank from challenge. "He does not have to ask permission [to perform risky surgery] because of our unique relationship. We trained him here and we know him."

Lee's expertise was kidney transplants, though. This was the area in which he and Mendez first worked. This surgery became so routine, Mendez got bored. He wanted more challenge. In 1984, Lee selected him to lead the surgical effort on liver transplants. "I knew he was the best," Lee would say later. "After all, I trained him." Lee scrubbed for the first several liver transplants, but rarely did so now. This case was special, however. Mendez wanted to run it by Lee.

They had an almost father-son relationship, born out of overcoming common prejudices. In addition, Mendez's European background went nicely with Lee's Oriental heritage, which placed great stress on respect for age and authority. Although by temperament quite different, the calm Asian and the fiery Spaniard shared an old-school respect for the student-teacher relationship, the wise old man and the younger disciple. As they stood in the vascular surgery offices in the Nelson Clinic, Dr. Lee asked again, "Why did you take this case, Jerry? It's a transplant after portacaval shunt and no one has ever survived such surgery. All of Starzl's patients died."

Mendez explained, "Both Carithers and I have told him that no one who previously had a portacaval shunt has come off the table alive after transplant surgery."

Lee reminded Mendez, "Starzl's a very aggressive guy. He is a very smart and a very good technical surgeon, so if he says he has serious doubts about the feasibility of a transplant after a portacaval shunt, we should take his hesitation very seriously."

Without shrinking, and brimming with confidence, Mendez explained, "I know insurance companies say, 'We will pay for this except if the patient has had a portacaval shunt.' Oh wow, this is just official company policy. But medically, the arteriogram indicates no problem and the portal vein and other veins are not so thrombosed that there is no hope of supplying the new liver with a good blood supply. So technically, then, a transplant can be done."

Growing more confident in his conversation with his mentor, Mendez asserted, "I can do it, I'm sure. It's a judgment call. Robbins' surgery is dramatic because it has written all over it, 'don't do this, don't do this . . . there is no question, don't do this.' Now when I say there is no question in my mind that we can do this, you know I mean I'm ninety percent sure. Everybody who has enough sense knows it could be difficult; it could be impossible or it could fall apart. But on the other hand, they also rationalize and think that it is surgically feasible.

"Gee," he continued with one of his few non-expletives, "I don't see any anatomical reason it can't be done. It may be very tough. But, if you do enough of them you are going to find a few that you can do. Several of them may be totally impossible because something will fall apart while you're doing it. But I can do this one."

Lee agreed.

o

The confident, macho surgeons joined with the nurturing Ann Reid Priest and Bob Carithers to complete a diverse team of health-care specialists and set the stage for my transplant. The yin and yang came together nicely in the MCV liver transplant team.

4

Friends

All men who have had an effect on the course of
human history, all of them without exception, were
capable and effective only because they were ready
to accept the inevitable.
Hermann Hesse, *Demian*

Now John Robbins, 47, is dying. At first it read just like another
newspaper article. I needed a few minutes to realize that the line
contained my name and described my condition. *How does it feel to die?*
As I read, the words spelled out in front of me in the newspaper made
everything seem more final, more certain.

The words were those of Polly Paddock, an old friend from
Charlotte and a columnist for the *Charlotte Observer*. She had learned
from my cousin that I was sick and in a lot of trouble, and she called me
in Fredericksburg to inquire about my health. We had a long talk
renewing an old friendship from the heady days of peace and rock and
roll in the sixties. She wrote about my dilemma in her next column. She
began, "His was one of the most familiar faces on the '60s scene in
Charlotte: a long-haired, outspoken UNCC history professor named John
Robbins. He attended peace rallies. Hosted a radio talk show. Narrowly
lost two political races: for the Charlotte City Council in 1971, the N.C.
House of Representatives in 1972. . . . Two years later, Robbins chucked
it all. He began an odyssey that took him to a Buddhist monastery in
Thailand for three years, back to Charlotte in 1980 . . . back to Bangkok
in 1983. . . ."

53

I'm reading my own obituary, I thought to myself. *How will I be remembered?* Various of Polly's words, scattered through her column, did, in a way, sum up my life: "long-haired; outspoken; peace activist; a Virginian with a Ph.D. from Rice University; energetic, brash, idealistic; involved in a wide array of liberal causes; an Episcopalian; a tenured professor."

The story gave the brief history of my illness, mentioned my Buddhist experience, explained my medical problem, and reported that I now found myself with no money to finance a transplant, my "only hope for life." It ended by quoting me: "There are efforts to make public financing for transplants available, but I can't wait. I feel like the last soldier to be shot before an armistice."

My life boiled down to twenty inches of newsprint. I asked myself: *How are lives summed up? How are people remembered? What are we remembered for? How can a listing of birth and death dates, cause of death, education, occupation, and survivors measure a human life? If they cannot, what else can? What does our life mean?*

This newspaper account of my impending demise led me to ponder what I had learned about life and death during the years I practiced Buddhism intensely as a monk at the Suan Mok Monastery in Thailand. I had spent hours with the abbot of my monastery, the Venerable Buddhadasa Bhikku, who explained much to me in an effort to allow me to come to my own understanding. As we sat in front of his dwelling in the quietude of a monastic, jungle environment, Buddhadasa often talked to me about Buddhist teachings on life and death. He tried to lead me to "see" that the two are inseparable.

Throughout my years in the monastery, I had explored pessimism and hope with my teachers. I began to find some assurance to counteract the despair about the world that had propelled me to the feet of Buddhadasa and the monks at the Suan Mok. I explained to the abbot that I wanted to believe this existence meant something. "What does our existence mean?" I asked the venerable master.

"Nothing," he responded indifferently. He expanded on his laconic answer by explaining that "nothing" in this case had two meanings. First, it implies that nothing of strictly material value is worth getting, and second, it means that nothing is worth being. He elaborated, " 'Getting' refers to setting one's heart on property, position, wealth, or any pleasing object, and 'being' refers to awareness of one's status as husband, wife, rich man, poor man, winner, loser."

"Is our existence, our life itself, then not worth setting our heart on?" I asked gently.

"No," he answered, "because we should not even set our hearts on the awareness of being oneself. If we can completely give up the idea of being oneself, then being oneself will no longer be the source of suffering. . . . The truth and struggle necessary to maintain one's state of being are simply the result of blind infatuation with things, of clinging to things."

Another scholarly old monk, Tan Mutti, acted as an additional inspiration for me. During the Pansa, a time in the year (July-October) when wandering stops and the monks spend the rainy months within the boundaries of the monastery, I passed hours with this distinguished old man mining his wealth of knowledge and breadth of insight. Once, he asked me about existentialism. We read Camus and Sartre together and examined two passages I had copied into my diary years before. From Camus (*The Stranger*):

And on a wide view I could see that it makes little difference whether one dies at the age of thirty or three score and ten— since in either case other men and women will continue living, the world will go on as before.

And from Sartre (*The Wall*):

A few hours or a few years of waiting are all the same when you've lost the illusion of being eternal.

The old monk pronounced these passages "Buddhism without hope."

My discussions with teachers like Buddhadasa and Tan Mutti, along with periods of intense meditation during solitary retreats at Koh Samui, an island off the East Coast of Thailand in the South China Sea, helped me clarify my understanding of life and death.

Bringing this understanding back to a Western and Christian world was difficult for me. I felt a need to explain myself to those who cared about me, but despite a lifetime in teaching, the ability to explain these things to others escaped me. I feared appearing indifferent, the great sin of the West and the sixties' culture ("If you're not part of the solution, then you're part of the problem"). I knew I had to choose my words carefully. I walked a thin line both outwardly and inwardly.

The Buddhist emphasis on nonattachment and the inevitability of death were now a part of me. It was the source of great comfort, because I had long been puzzled that the Christian tradition also taught the inevitability of death, but then seemed to deny it in a message of overwhelming concern with some kind of future life in a place called "heaven." I discovered that most Americans do not like to talk about death. For many, it is a morbid subject. To look at death, to acknowledge its reality, to affirm its inevitability, to confirm and talk about it did not seem morbid to me, however. Why were people so jumpy about the subject? Perhaps, I reasoned, it is because of a macho, "fight for life" belief that seems to pervade the culture. Whatever the answer, I found myself caught in a bind between asking others to help save my life and talking about my acceptance of death. I did not want to send the wrong signal to people. "Why help him if he already accepts death?" I was locked inside myself. It seemed a cruel choice.

My family and friends reduced my dilemma to insignificance. They did not see my acceptance of death as an excuse not to help. While I wanted to face the world alone, I also began to draw strength from their strength. Initially, my greatest fear was that people would believe my life represented a rejection of their values and would conclude, "He chose to wander, now let him face the consequence of his actions." Perhaps my fears rose from my belief that one should be prepared to accept the consequence of one's own actions. As a result, I was quite willing to accept what had happened to me. Yet no matter how much I said, "I am prepared to accept my consequences or fate," I still wanted to live. My philosophy, my experience, had not altered in any significant way that desire. I only wanted the same thing I had always wanted, that is to live in a way that made this moment count—not becoming too preoccupied with either past or present. The present is all that counts. It is all we truly have. Consequently, any struggle for life had to be conducted in the present moment. It cannot be conducted in some brave or courageous focus elsewhere. That would not be consistent with my belief that living in the face of adversity is not courageous or heroic, but natural.

I underestimated my friends. They wanted—were willing—to help. But I found it very difficult to ask people for help. Earlier I told Ray Wallace, my close friend from college days at Hampden-Sydney, "A transplant is my only hope. I don't have the money, and I can't ask." Without a moment's hesitation, he responded, "You can't, but we can."

And he and others did. Ray, along with fraternity brother Bill Ware, a teacher in Richmond, and classmate Lew Drew, currently Dean of Students at Hampden-Sydney College, launched a campaign to raise money from college friends. Mary Jo Doherty, a high-school classmate now living in Ithaca, New York, where her husband was on the faculty at Cornell, wrote all the members of our 1956 class at Haverling Central School in Bath, New York. Friends from graduate school at Rice University did the same with a group who had studied history together and now were on faculties in universities around the country. Several colleagues from my days at the University of North Carolina and Queens College in Charlotte contacted old friends and students from my teaching days. Because I objected to the obscene media events that fund drives can become, my friends limited their effort to a single letter.

While my friends were contacting one another, I felt much more comfortable trying to change the system. I turned Retta's front porch into my office and began a letter-writing campaign, doing so with all the zeal I had employed in the other causes of my life. The task of challenging the system spurred me to action and, for the time being, deflected my thoughts from the apparent hopelessness of my situation. Changing your life and waiting passively for the end is as destructive as denial itself when you face death.

Because states administer Medicaid, I directed my campaign at state officials. Virginia stubbornly remained one of only sixteen states refusing funds for liver transplants, as the Virginia Medicaid Board insisted upon labeling the procedure "experimental." The Board even cited statistics purporting to demonstrate a low success rate for liver transplants, though no other agency or medical group ever verified the Board's figures. Surely, I reasoned, this was a short-sighted policy. Obviously no one had ever presented a good case to the Board.

I gathered evidence to show the bureaucracy the error of its ways. Reason would surely prevail in such a vital issue, I thought. I sent carefully crafted letters to major state officials, including Governor Gerald Baliles, Secretary of Human Resources Eva Tieg, Director of

Medical Assistance Service Ray Sorrell, and Director of Medical Support Robert Wood. My position seemed so reasonable, I was certain these people would respond favorably. I developed fact-sheets on liver transplantation and success rates. I quoted from conferences, reports. I wrote the officials that the nature of liver disease made it impossible for me to work or to obtain private insurance. I asked the officials to make an exception to the state policy that denied Medicaid funding for liver transplants, because the transplant held out the possibility that I could return "to the ranks of independent, self-sustaining taxpaying citizens."

On a beautiful July day I got my answer. It came in the form of a letter from Robert L. Wood, M.D., Director of Medical Support. I tore open the envelope and read eagerly. By the third paragraph, I began to slide down in my seat as despair swept over me. *Why go on?* I thought to myself. The letter contained stereotypical answers from a bureaucracy. Dr. Wood wrote, ". . . Since liver transplants for adults is [sic] generally considered to be experimental, I have no choice but to deny your request for exception to this policy. . . ."

I wanted to scream, but I was quiet. I struggled to regain my center.

Not all public officials, however, responded so coolly. Former North Carolina Attorney General Rufus Edmisten, State Senator Bobby Scott of Newport News, and Delegate Bill Wilson of Covington (a long-time member of the House of Delegates and college classmate) contacted the Governor and various agencies in the state government to see what could be done. Local Democratic activist Jim Gibbs arranged a meeting for me attended by Secretary of Human Resources Eva Teig; a representative from the Governor's Office, Pat Lambeth; and the Director of Medical Assistance Services, Ray Sorrell. The bureaucrats were duly sympathetic, but said nothing could be done because the legislature had not made funds available to allow Medicaid to fund liver transplants.

The issue also gained national attention in the summer of 1986. Tennessee Senator Albert Gore, Jr., led the fight. I contacted Senator Gore's office for information and encouragement. From his early days in the House, Gore labored for both adequate funding for transplants and for a national system to match donors and recipients. After holding hearings, he sponsored the National Organ Transplant Act, which among other things ended the practice of buying and selling organs and established a national computer system to match donors and recipients.

His legislation (The National Organ Transplant Act of 1985) sailed through Congress, but ran into Reagan Administration opposition. While the president hesitated, people died. Reagan, looking duly sympathetic, satisfied himself with photo opportunities on the White House lawn appealing for an organ for a dying child at the same time his aides blocked the implementation of Gore's bill.

I followed the fight with growing interest. Senator Gore spoke for people like me when he declared that organ transplants should not be limited to the wealthy or to those who could mount the most effective publicity campaign. Such campaigns for children were all right, but I felt they were an especially cruel burden for an adult to endure. I did not want my life to end in a circus of publicity, of bake sales and car washes. *Can't I die with some dignity?* I often asked myself.

I counted myself fortunate because my friends' campaign was relatively low-key, with only two newspaper articles in Charlotte and Richmond. Ultimately, Ray Wallace, the director of my fundraising campaign, formalized the earlier agreements that would allow me to go on the waiting list for a liver after raising $20,000 and promising to make a good-faith effort to secure the remainder. Unofficially, the hospital agreed that if I survived, I would not have to begin a new life hundreds of thousands of dollars in debt. The arrangement both heartened and disturbed me. I knew that my chance for life came because of my background, education, and friends. I felt guilty because I knew that if I had not gone to the right schools and known influential people, none of this would have happened. I wanted to live. I remained quiet.

My friends, however, provided a far more important service for me than money-raising in the summer of 1986. They cared and took the trouble to contact me. I got telephone calls and letters from friends all over the world, wishing me well and making offers of support. My students, now spread across the country, wrote to reminisce and to update me on their lives and careers. (Many had received a copy of Polly Paddock's column in the *Charlotte Observer*, sent by their parents who still lived in the Charlotte area.) Several who were rock music fans and fellow political and peace activists gathered in Savannah, Georgia, called, and sent me a souvenir T-shirt after a Moody Blues' concert. Many others—including a large number of women who returned to the university after their children were in school—wrote to tell how me I had helped them in their student days and beyond. Some were carrying on the tradition, and now they, too, were teachers. Hearing from students and friends reassured and strengthened my resolve. They helped me cast away lingering doubt about my life and find balance and right effort for that which lay ahead.

5

Waiting

*His statement to himself should have been, 'I possess
this now therefore am happy,' instead of what it so
Victorianly was, 'I cannot possess this forever and therefore
am sad.'*
John Fowles, *The French Lieutenant's Woman*

7 August

Retta and I are preparing for one of our frequent trips to Richmond during this hot, sultry Virginia summer of 1986. Today, however, is special. I will officially make the down payment for the liver. Exactly one month ago, Rev. Charles Sydnor and the vestry at Retta's and Jay's church established the St. George's Medical Fund in order to collect money to aid my transplant. Substantial contributions from church programs established to aid men in need launched the drive. Vestrymen, friends in Fredericksburg, and family quickly subscribed the sufficient amount for the required $20,000 to put me on the waiting list for the transplant. The speed with which this was accomplished surprised me. I was thankful that my friends had been able to spare me a longer, more tortuous wait to get on the list. Nevertheless, we still had much more money to raise.

After picking up the check from the administrator of the fund, I said to Retta as I folded myself into her ancient MGB, "You know, this check is for more than the mortgage on the first house I bought in 1969. Sort of odd to think that my liver is going to cost more than my first house."

We headed to Richmond to meet Ray Wallace for lunch at the

Country Club of Virginia. The Club, with its columned portico, eighteenth-century furniture, and subservient waiters is the symbol of old Virginia values and the heart of the conservative Virginia tradition, which is now giving way to the realities of the New Dominion. I quipped over lunch, "The Directors might lift your membership, Ray, if they knew you were entertaining Medicaid recipients in their club!"

"You can't stop, can you, John? You never let up. Healthy or sick you're always crusading. You damned liberals are all alike," Ray snapped back.

We were only continuing as usual. I always tried to tease Ray, a died-in-the-wool Goldwater/Reagan Republican who has remained one of my closest friends since college when we both tried to bait professors and administrators. Our exchange this day at the club showed that our relationship was continuing as normally as possible despite the fact that I was facing death and that he was trying desperately through fundraising to stave off what I regarded as inevitable.

Retta, a silent witness to this little exchange, was initially surprised at our conversation. On the drive from the Club to my appointment at the hospital, I explained to her I had discovered the importance of reaching the right balance between stiff-upper-lip perseverance and grim resignation. In difficult times, friendship is best maintained as it always has been. Nothing is gained by focusing on impending death, nor is anything gained by denying what is almost certain to happen. These times require a subtle balance between acceptance and non-acceptance. If the person facing death sends the right signals, friends will follow along naturally.

Arriving at the hospital, I had another talk with Dr. Carithers about the seriousness of my condition. Then, Ann Reid came in the room carrying a little black box, my beeper to alert me when a donor liver became available. "We'll always try to call you first. So only turn this on when you are out of telephone range; then keep it on and with you at all times." I took the beeper, wrote the numbers to call in response, and stared at it. I was waiting for someone to die in order that I might live, an unpleasant thought that I immediately dismissed. Nevertheless, the beeper became my lifeline. From this moment on, I knew any sound from it or any telephone call might be my last. From that moment, I lived tethered to my telephone lifeline. The wait, the excruciating wait, began. The wait can dominate your life, turn you testy, nasty, edgy, and totally self-centered. It is, to say the least, not a pleasant time.

Rick Liverman, the social worker, arrived next and took me to pay for my liver. I got my receipt. I looked at it lying limply in my hand and slowly realized I held the most essential receipt of my life—a receipt for a chance to live. I wondered how I might ever come to place a value on the number of dollars that receipt represented. *How much should a chance to live cost?* I asked myself.

With financial considerations taken care of for the time being, Ann wanted us to focus on what to expect with the transplant. Those in charge of MCV's liver transplant program wanted both patients and their families to understand the course of treatment. Carithers and Priest spent a great amount of time explaining things to me, because, in Carithers' words, "surgeons don't do a particularly good job informing and educating people about operations." Ann then scheduled a visit to the Medical Respiratory Intensive Care Unit (the MRICU), where liver and kidney transplant patients return after surgery. As Ret and I toured the MRICU on the fourth floor of MCV's main hospital, the calm, cool efficiency of the place scared me. Machines, monitors, and eerie sounds filled the room. Despite life-and-death stakes, everything moved at an almost relaxed pace, and everyone appeared under control. The nurse in charge explained to Retta what I would look like after surgery, with sixteen lines and drains in my body.

Following the trip to the ICU came an explanation of the operation. We read MCV's consent form for liver transplant surgery. "I have had a complete evaluation of my liver disease. From the results of this evaluation, I understand that there is no known cure for my liver disease and that my liver disease will ultimately be fatal. I also understand that a transplant operation is technically feasible."

"Yes, I understand that," I told Ann Reid. "No questions."

We continued reading. "I am fully aware that I have only a 60% chance of surviving the operation and the first three months following surgery. The major risk during surgery is from severe bleeding that cannot be stopped. [Previous surgery, the portacaval shunt, made this an even more severe threat in my case.] Following surgery there is a continued risk of internal bleeding and infections. Because of these complications I understand that there is a high likelihood that I may need an additional operation."

"John,' said Ann Reid evenly, "you realize, according to what Dr. Mendez has already told you, your chances are not as good as those mentioned in this form. The portacaval shunt lowers your odds considerably. As yet, we do not know of anyone who has survived a transplant after a shunt operation."

"Yes, that has been made quite clear to me."

Next, we read about all the likely side-effects of medication and confinement in the ICU. "Following surgery I will be in an intensive care unit for at least two to four weeks. I will be on an artificial ventilator to help me breathe. During this time I may be in some pain and I may be deprived of sleep because of the nursing care and many tests that may be needed for my care. I may develop a severe infection, bleeding or kidney failure. In addition, I may become confused because of the medications I am given. Finally, there is continuing risk that my body may reject the transplanted liver. In the event of these complications I may have to undergo biopsies of my liver and lung. If kidney failure occurs, I may need treatment with an artificial kidney. It is also possible that I may have to undergo additional operations for bleeding, infection or damage to my bile ducts.

"I will have to stay in the hospital for at least three months following surgery. There will be continued risk of infection, rejection of the liver and blockage of my bile ducts. These complications may require me to undergo biopsies of the liver or lung and possibly an additional operation."

And finally, we looked at the long-term implications of the transplant. "From the time the new liver is transplanted into my body until the end of my life, I will have to take two medications, prednisone and cyclosporine, to keep my body from destroying the new liver. Prednisone may result in weight gain with fullness of face and shoulders, acne, continued risk of serious infections, thinning of my bones with possible bone collapse and diabetes requiring insulin injection. Cyclosporine can cause kidney failure, which may require treatment with an artificial kidney for a short period. In addition this new drug can cause high blood pressure, an increase in facial and body hair, an increase in the size of my gums and non-cancerous breast lumps. The long-term risks of this medication are not known. I am aware that cyclosporine is also very expensive, costing almost $4,000 per year. . . ."

"Wow! That's a lot. I'll be going from expensive surgery to an expensive lifelong drug therapy. Will I ever get off the drugs?"

"No! At this time, these drugs are a lifetime commitment."

Then we finished reading. "I have considered the major psychological and financial burdens that may result both for me and my family from having this operation."

She looked at me. "Any questions, John?"

"None, thanks. I understand everything." I failed, however, to take sufficient notice that a majority of the consent form dealt with post-operative problems. I overlooked these complications in my eagerness to get on with surgery. Most people—and I was no exception—always focus on the operation, believing that if you survive the operation, the real problem is over. Everyone is cautioned that problems for a transplant patient really begin after surgery, but the warning never takes hold. There is no way it can.

"You will have to sign this form as part of the pre-op preparations, before the surgery, when we call you in after we have located a suitable liver," Ann concluded.

Ret and I returned to Fredericksburg and our lives would never be the same again.

I was on a list waiting for a liver transplant. I got up in the middle of the night to turn off my beeper. I had forgotten to do so before going to bed. I had not yet established my rhythm of living and waiting. As I discovered in the days ahead, the wait is always with you. Before doing even the simplest task or taking the shortest trip from the house, you question yourself: *Do you think you should be doing this now? Perhaps the liver will come. The beeper won't work and the doctors will give the liver to someone else.* I was scared to stay away from home for long periods of time. The wait even does strange things to your friends.

"John, I just heard about a big accident on I-95. Have you heard anything from MCV yet about a liver?"

"No, Janet, it can't happen that fast, but thanks for caring."

The wait, THE WAIT, consumes life. The trick is not to let it control your conduct, although it is always in your mind. I tried exercises I had previously learned in meditation to stay focused. Sometimes making a joke of the whole process is good. One of my friends who shared my sometimes dark sense of humor thought we could have a lottery in which people would guess the time and date I would get the transplant. You'll do almost anything—including dark humor—to get your mind off the wait.

22 August

Another appointment with Dr. Carithers. "Everything's okay, John. Your numbers look good." Which meant that the values measured in blood tests I took biweekly showed that the liver was still functioning, the blood count was still good.

"When do you think we'll have the operation?"

"There's just no way of telling. It could be any time. We never know." These assurances worked. My trust level remained high. The hours that Carithers had previously spent talking with me about everything from literature to basketball and medicine now paid off. I needed to trust him, and he needed my trust in order to help me. This mutually shared trust, like faith in spiritual life, is essential to hope and cure.

29 August

Three of my college classmates were quoted in a Richmond *News Leader* story about Hampden-Sydney rallying to help a long-ago graduate who had lived a life somewhat different from the Hampden-Sydney norm. The quotes pretty much covered the range of friends' responses.

From Ray Wallace, the political emphasis: "It has been an educational experience, no question about it. I think maybe we are a little more sensitized that something has to be done, and a lot of us are in positions where we can be heard."

From Lewis Drew, the philosophical: "He's a very sensitive, intelligent person who just had the strength of his convictions. . . . His life itself could be an example that might not result in product, but instead might be oriented toward values and reflection."

From Bill Wilson, a member of the House of Delegates, with whom friendship was based on the intimacy that is part of attending a small college where all students know one another: "We weren't big buddies or anything. But it's a classmate. It's a real personal thing. He's in trouble, and somebody calls and asks, 'Will you help?' And it was satisfying and personal, and that's all."

1 September

Recalling my fear of the machines in the hospital, I sign the Virginia Natural Death Act, with instructions to place it in my medical records:

> If at any time I should have a terminal condition and my attending physician has determined that there is no reasonable expectation of recovery from such condition and my death is imminent, where the application of life-prolonging procedures would serve only to artificially prolong the dying process, I direct that such procedures be withheld or withdrawn, and that I be permitted to die naturally with only the administration of medication or the performance of any medical procedure deemed necessary to provide me with comfort or to alleviate pain.

7 September

The wait reaches one month. I go today to see Charles Sydnor, the priest at St. George's Church. As I settle into the chair at his office, I explain, "Charles, Retta wants some kind of memorial service and there are a few things I would like. First, I want two folk songs 'Turn, Turn, Turn,' which contains verses from *Ecclesiastes*, and Woody Guthrie's 'This Land Is Your Land.' I have already marked passages from Thoreau and the *Dhammapada* [part of Buddhist scripture] that I believe might be appropriate. Then whatever you think would be suitable as comforting prayers for Retta and the others. That would be totally up to you. After all, the service is for them."

We searched the Episcopal *Book of Common Prayer* and put together what I thought was a quite acceptable service. I thanked him and walked home.

This session with Rev. Sydnor concluded my preparations for death. I had no financial settlements to make. The illness had bankrupted me. Waiting remained my lone task.

12 September

Dr. Carithers emphasizes, and I agree, that my life should remain as absolutely normal as possible. Janet Payne involves me in the Congressional race in Virginia's First District, where she is a coordinator of the district for State Senator Bobby Scott. Tonight she takes me to a fundraiser at the Fredericksburg Country Club. I enjoy the evening tremendously.

22 September

"St. George's Medical Fund. Dear Friends, Enclosed is our check to you, which is the tithe from our E.Y.C. [Episcopal Young Churchmen] budget. I hope this will help further your cause in the name of our Lord. With warmest wishes from our E.Y.C." [of St. John's, Charlotte]

Few letters pleased me more. The current advisor to the group had been a member of the E.Y.C. when my wife and I were advisors from 1969 to 1971.

23 September

Donn Waldron, a traveling companion from my wandering days in Southeast Asia, called from California. Since my return from Bangkok, he had called periodically to see how I was doing.

"I would love to see you again, John."

"Well, Donn," I replied, hoping not to sound too dramatic, yet trying to give an accurate assessment of where I was. "I don't know what to tell you, but if that's what you mean, you had better come soon. I don't know how much time I have left."

"I'll fly back East for your birthday. How's that?"

"I'd love that. I'm looking forward to it."

25 September

Donn arrived from L.A. to celebrate my birthday. We talk mainly about good times in the past: meeting on the boat going to Samosir Island in Indonesia, tramping around the Malay peninsula with a group of international travelers we called the alphabet people, exchanging visits in L.A., Charlotte, and Bangkok.

28 September

My forty-eighth and, what I am sure is, my final birthday. You sum up a life when you think it is your last birthday. I had no regrets. I reflected on a classmate's question the previous July at our thirtieth high-school reunion. "Are you angry?" he asked. "No," I answered without much hesitation, though with a little surprise.

I wasn't angry then. I am not angry now. I had never been angry. Frustrated at times, but not angry. I never felt, as I heard some who faced certain death tell reporters, that "it's so unfair." No, it's not. It's only *chun nun eng*—just the way things are. It's not unfair. It's not blind fate. It's not bad luck. I never passed through what the pop psychologists tell us are the stages of preparing for death, from denial to acceptance. Neither of those words, nor any in between, ever described how I felt. All of those stages seem to suggest a victim, and I did not feel like a victim. Victims die. I wanted to live, but not in a way that made me a victim.

How could I ever explain it? When you maintain a *chun nun eng*, or that's-just-the-way-things-are, attitude, you avoid the "Why me?" questions, which are extraordinarily destructive. In addition, you avoid falling into the trap of trying to bargain, another counter-productive course for terminally ill people. I said to myself that I would not change one decision in my life even if could have foreseen the consequences of my actions. I quickly realized that such speculation was yet another kind of self-defeating trap. I picked up a book I had read in many stages of my life. I turned the well-worn pages of *Walden,* and my eyes fell on one of my favorite passages (one expressing an attitude toward life that I, too, had tried to embrace):

> I went to the woods because I wished to live deliberately, to front only the essential facts of life, and see if I could not learn what it had to teach, and not, when I came to die, discover that I had not lived. I did not wish to live what was not life, living is so dear; nor did I wish to practice resignation, unless it was quite necessary.

Sometimes I felt like a reincarnated Thoreau, especially when I recalled my three years of a Walden-like existence in a small hut in the jungles of Thailand and when I remembered that he, too, had died at a young age. I closed my Thoreau and considered some verses from the Buddhist's *Vissudhimagga* or *Path of Purification,* which I had copied long ago in my diary:

Nirvana is, but not the man who seeks it. [and] The path exists, but not the traveler on it.

I also read some verses that Jeff Meyer, a Quaker and a professor of religion at UNCC, had sent me, saying that they were the best expression of his feelings about death:

Your mind-essence is not subject to birth or death. It is neither being nor nothingness, neither emptiness nor form-and-color. Nor is it something that feels pain or joy. However much you try to know [with your rational mind] that which is now sick, you cannot. Yet if you think of nothing, wish for nothing, want to understand nothing, cling to nothing, and only ask yourself, "What is the true substance of the Mind of this one who is now suffering?" ending your days like clouds fading in the sky, you will eventually be freed from your painful bondage to endless change.

Finally, I sought to put my feelings into words. I wrote:

"Sickness enables me to feel what I previously knew, but did not understand: the unimportance and meaninglessness of my own existence. The 'my' creates a self, an egoistic existence which leads to unwise feelings, wants, attachments, and clinging thereby giving rise to suffering. The self exists only as a product of our own mind. Feeling reveals our world of 'my's' as a sham existence. Existence itself is not meaningless; 'my' makes existence meaningless. Feeling allows one to see that a paradox is not at all paradoxical.

"As a result, unable to feel, many ask questions about future life out of a misunderstanding of existence. 'My,' in combination with existence, produces undue concern with the future, 'my future existence,' 'my future life.' When one realizes and feels the non-existence of 'my,' the question of future life sinks into non-importance. In cultures overwhelmed with time, life after death attracts unnecessary attention when, in fact, it is rather unimportant. Some pre-eminently concerned with their own existence, therefore, place primary importance on heaven ('my' continuing existence) and never feel. They fall back on moral codes emphasizing and distorting rules out of all proportion, producing neurotic, guilt-ridden people. One can only feel in a Zen or Taoist way. You can't define 'feel' because when you do, you don't feel. And if you can define 'feel,' you don't feel. If you feel, you don't need a definition. Those who know don't tell, and those who tell don't know.

"I am not sad. I am not happy. I am not resigned. I just am."

2 October

"How much longer Dr. Carithers?" I ask.

"We don't know, John. Your numbers continue to look good. You are doing all right for now."

Doubt begins to rise ever so subtly in my mind. I try to ignore it. For the moment I am successful. "See you in two weeks or sooner," I say hopefully as I leave his office.

7 October

Letters from students, activists, and friends continue to sustain me as the wait enters its second agonizing month.

17 October

"Dr. Carithers, I feel terrible. I know I am getting worse. Are you trying to find me a liver or not? Do you really plan to transplant me?"

"Yes, John. So far your numbers look good."

I am rather tired of this answer. "It's been over two months. What's happening?"

"We're looking, John, but remember you are a special case. We want all the surgeons here because of the difficulties involving the portacaval shunt. Dr. Mendez prefers a local donor so he doesn't have to worry with all the inherent difficulties involved in a long-distance recovery. He wants to control as many factors as possible. Distance, airplane schedules, the other hospital's schedule, weather—all complicate his timing. Your surgery already presents enough complications."

Carithers placates me again. I decide to press my luck and ask him one more thing that had been on my mind. "Dr. Carithers," I begin, pointing to the strings on my wrists, "these pieces of string on each of my wrists are called *sai sila,* which is literally translated as 'line of the teaching or rules.' I know to most people they look just like another piece of string, but they have an important meaning in Buddhism. I have a special connection to them because a friend put them on me in a very tense time. The Thai doctors and nurses knew what they were and didn't cut them off. The strings survived the portacaval shunt, and I have become attached to them. Do you think they would interfere with the transplant or cause any undue problems? I'd like to keep them on."

A broad smile lit up his face, "Of course, John. We don't want to challenge the gods!"

"Well, it's not exactly like that, but I have acquired a rather strong faith in them," I explained.

"I understand," he replied. "I'll mention it to Ann Reid."

"Thanks." And I never gave it much thought again.

31 October

I am not in a very good mood when I walk into Dr. Carithers' office. "Well, we're headed for three months, and I am getting worse. I am not going to make it to the transplant at this rate."

He tries to reassure me. "John, I know it's tough waiting, and many people at this stage think they are forgotten, but we have not forgotten you. We're still looking."

"Who makes the decision on when I get transplanted?"

"That is ultimately Dr. Mendez's decision, and he is very picky about what livers he will take. It is not at all unusual for him to refuse a liver that another center will take. Remember, the worst thing that can happen to you is for the liver not to work. In your condition, you're only going to get one shot at it. It's going to have to be 'go' all the way the first time. There will be no second chance for you. That's why we have to be so careful."

Once again the straightforward approach of Dr. Carithers works. I am reassured again, and we shift the conversation to basketball and North Carolina. "John, you'll see Carolina play again. I promise."

I return to Fredericksburg feeling better. Retta had arranged a Halloween party that night to boost my spirits, and it did. I made a note in my diary: "Fun costumes, and fun people . . . a good time."

I was following Dr. Carithers' advice to keep my life as normal as possible. I went to art shows and plays at Mary Washington College with Retta. Janet and I continued to work together as Bobby Scott's run for Congress was nearing its climax. The election was only five days away.

12 November

As the wait enters its fourth month, the cast of ABC's "All My Children" soap opera learns of my condition, and today I receive a large package. I tear it open to find a script and autographed pictures of most of the cast, including some of my favorites like Tad and Erica. I am delighted and particularly amused with the note of Peter Bergman, who plays Dr. Cliff Warner. He writes, "John, No matter how bad it gets remember at least Cliff Warner is not your doctor!" Soaps become the center of my life, as I am no longer able to sustain much reading and writing. My fatigue is becoming more of a problem each day.

My days are spent hanging on. Retta fixes my breakfast and lunch and leaves the food in the refrigerator before going to school. Getting up, washing, brushing my teeth, putting in my contacts, and eating breakfast usually exhausts me for the day. I can still handle the soaps despite the tangled web of relationships. Good is still good. Evil remains evil. And despite momentary evidence to the contrary, bad is punished.

Ret usually finds me asleep when she gets home from school. Awakened from my lethargy, I join her in watching "General Hospital," as she too becomes hooked on all the machinations of Port Charles. She tries to coax me out to the movies or to art shows or shopping, but usually I beg off because my energy level is so low.

14 November

Another appointment with Dr. Carithers, and another round of "We're not sure, but . . .your numbers are good." On my way to the lab for some blood tests, I bump into psychologist Mary Ellen Olbrisch, who is making a brief visit to the clinic from the psychology clinic three floors above. I can tell from the shocked expression on her face that I must look very bad.

"How are you, John?" she inquires.

"Not too good, Mary Ellen. I've just come from Dr. Carithers, and he says my numbers are good, but I'm not sure. I surely feel like I am declining, and I don't think I am going to make it to the transplant." I can see from the look on her face that she agrees with me, not with Dr. Carithers.

17 November

News of my decline is now circulating widely among my friends in many parts of Thailand. "Dear John, We are so sorry to hear that you are very sick. The money we sent is a small gift, but we want you to know that you have friends in Thailand and we always remember you." It is signed by eleven members of the English Department at Srinakharinwirot University Prasarnmitr, where I last taught in Bangkok.

20 November

Ray Wallace drives up from Richmond to take me to dinner. "John, have they told you any more about getting that liver?"

"No, Ray. Dr. Carithers says they are trying, but nothing has come about yet. He says my numbers are okay, but I don't feel like they are good. I think I am declining." From the look on his face and his questions, I understand that Ray feels there is almost no hope. I know he is angry at MCV. Trying not to sound despondent, I tell him, "I will keep you informed. But I've almost reached four months, and I just don't know. Please always know how much I appreciate your friendship and all that everyone has done for me." Ray helps me back to the car, takes me home. Silence thunders at our parting.

15 December

The Christmas season approaches, but I really don't have the energy to pay much attention to the upcoming times of joy and birth right now. I make plans for Christmas, though, and Ret takes me shopping. Here, my growing confusion—which I first noticed when I found it difficult to count my money and make change when buying goods—has been compounded by the confusion that being in a crowd of people produces in me. I am too puzzled to be able to do much. Christmas time, since my divorce and the death of my father and mother, has always been a difficult period for me because it is a family time, one I associate with the happiness of childhood.

This season points out to me more clearly than any other the consequences of living a wandering and solitary life. I continue in adulthood to expect the Christmas joy of youth, and am, of course, naturally let down. Dreams rarely conform to reality. Anticipation results in frustration. I know this with my mind, but do not feel it with my heart, and therefore do not truly understand. The separation of mind and heart always throws me into depression. I seem unable to do anything about it. My Christmas depression is an excellent illustration of the trap of anticipation. Anticipation is especially dangerous for one waiting for a transplant or for any major operation, because as the doctors explain—but you never realize or feel—it makes any postoperative time more difficult.

18 December

Retta goes with me to Dr. Carithers. I believe Retta is losing faith and is depressed. After all, these times must be very difficult on any family member. But it is hard for the sick person to empathize with the sorrow of family and friends because, *after all, I am the one who is dying.*

Illness often destroys relationships. We, the sick, have a tendency to forget others' sorrow while we are in the midst of our own. I don't know what else to do but to seem cheerful and not let her think I am losing faith in Dr. Carithers and MCV. I am, I realize, only following a pattern I developed in childhood and adolescence, when I always wanted to shield my parents from my hurt and my concerns, lest they be worried.

"What should we look for, Doctor?" Retta quizzes Dr. Carithers. "How do we know when he is so sick he should come to the hospital?"

"There is not one specific thing for you to look for at this moment, Retta. His fatigue and confusion do not seem to be out of proportion to his sickness. John is all right at home now. All our tests, at this point, show no particular cause for immediate alarm. John needs a transplant. We know that, and we are working on it. Just continue what you are doing."

I think he pacifies her for the time being. She doesn't want to worry me, and I don't want to worry her.

"John," Carithers says looking me directly in the eye, "I think your transplant will be soon. Mendez saw you bouncing off the wall the last time you were here and he has moved you to absolute number one on our waiting list."

25 December

I really don't remember much about the holiday season. Things are getting blurry and hazy to me. I sit down and just fall asleep.

28 December

Perhaps it's the holiday season, but the wait seems to be taking a toll. A smothering feeling of helplessness seems to grip everyone involved in my transplant wait. How to explain my feeling still eludes me. Perhaps words are not necessary. If I continue to express optimism, while at the same time maintaining an attitude of acceptance, those around will probably follow my lead. I try, but it's hard.

31 December

Usually on New Year's Eve, I try to imagine where I will be on the last day of the new year about to begin. Until I left the United States in 1974, this was an easy task, because my life followed a predictable pattern. Since 1974, however, New Year's Eve had found me in a host of different places—Bang Saen, Bangkok, Charlotte, Suan Mok, Hong Kong. I was never quite sure where I would be. It had made the last twelve years fun, exciting, vital. I didn't play the game this year.

9 January 1987

"Dr. Carithers, it was five months day before yesterday that I went on the waiting list. I've declined. I don't care what your numbers say. I'm weaker and physically nearer death. I know that. Do we have to look at the ethics of this situation? Am I such a high-risk patient, with such a low probability of success, that I am very low on the list and realistically will not get a liver? I certainly can understand a decision based on those criteria. I cannot accept one based on money, but I can on ethics and on medical probability. Maybe doctors think transplanting me will involve using a liver that might better be used for another person."

"John, you would not be taking a liver from anyone, so rest assured on that. You are long-shot for success, as we have already discussed on many occasions, but you will not take a liver from a better prospect."

"Then, Dr. Carithers, how do you select?"

"We don't make any other kinds of ethical judgments. The only thing we care about is compliance—in other words, will you take your medicine regularly and follow the proper diet, which will be necessary to keep you in good health. I don't care about your philosophy. I don't care about whether you're going to be a productive citizen or whether your life has more worth than any other—I think these are irrelevant. Who am I to judge? Who's to judge quality of life? Whether you're deserving of an organ? The only thing that we look at, from a very practical standpoint, is compliance. Are you going to take your medicine?

"The difficulty of the whole transplant process is the inability to predict an outcome in an individual case. Some people who seem medically to be better risks simply do not make it through the process. The ability to predict in individual situations is very, very, very poor. Thus, this long wait is not based on an either ethical considerations or any predictions we have made as to the probable outcome."

Once again his frankness calms me. The doctor provides a model on whom I can base my own attempts to steady worried friends and tell them that all will work out.

22 January

Fredericksburg and Richmond are hit with a major winter storm. Over a foot of snow closes road, stores, schools, and airports for the second time in a week. I have an appointment with Dr. Carithers, but cannot get down to Richmond because of the snow. Now I understand the difficulty of timing for a long-distance retrieval. Weather like today's would severely hamper any transplant attempt. But suppose there were no other choice?

30 January

I am having such difficulty with the daily routine of life now that Retta packs my bag when I leave for my postponed appointment with Dr. Carithers. She is convinced that once he sees me, he will put me in the hospital. Ret, the person most responsible for my day-to-day care, watches me deteriorate before her eyes. We play a little game with each other. I try very hard to be unconcerned, but yet not reach the point of resignation. I don't want to worry her or to make her sad. She in turn tries not to show her alarm at my condition and her increasing anger at MCV for not operating on me sooner.

I begin my visit with Dr. Carithers by asking, "Should I stay in the hospital now? I'm getting worse. I hate to run up the expense by waiting in the hospital, but I can't do much for myself now. I can hardly feed myself, much less prepare any food on my own. I am almost totally dependent on others."

"Hang on, John. You are still close to a hospital with good medical care right in Fredericksburg. We think it's better—if at all possible—for you to wait at home."

11 February

At dinner, Ret asks, "John, you're not eating your baked potato. It doesn't have too much protein. You always eat your baked potato. What's wrong?"

"I just don't feel too good, Ret. Don't worry."

She continues, "I want to go to the movies tonight. It's the Wednesday night dollar night. Do you want to go?"

"No, I don't feel like it. Besides there's a Carolina game on TV tonight I want to watch."

"I won't be long. Jay's on call, but Joan is home if you need anything."

After some time passes, I look up to see Retta again. She's back. "Oh, hi Retta. How was the movie?"

"We didn't get in. We got there too late. All the tickets were sold."

Ret was still in the room with me when, about fifteen minutes later, I turned and asked her, "Did you enjoy the movie?"

"We couldn't get a ticket and we didn't see the movie. Didn't I explain that to you just a few minutes ago?"

My ability to stay alert and keep track of what was going on around me forced Ret to spend a lot of time re-explaining things to me.

"I guess you did. I must have had one of my moments when I just blanked out and forgot the passage of time, although I'm afraid it's more than just forgetting. I'm just completely out of it some times. I can't remember what you say, because I'm just not here."

I insisted I knew what was going on, but I dozed off so frequently I was unaware that my beloved Tarheels were coasting to victory.

"Do you want me to turn off the TV before I go to bed?" Retta asked in the midst of one of my lapses.

"No, I'll do it. I want to watch the news after the game. Good night, Ret."

"Good night, John."

Part II

deLIVERance

For everything, there is a season and a time for every matter under heaven . . .

– Ecclesiastes 3:1

1

...a time to be born, a time to die...

Thursday, 12 February, 6:00 A.M.

Retta thinks to herself, *John didn't eat well last night . . . He was so confused. I'd better check on him before I go to school. I'm not sure he can stay by himself anymore. I think I may have to find someone to stay with him. I'll just take a look at him.*

The room smells just like death as Retta opens the door to make her check before going into the kitchen to start her coffee. The scene is hauntingly similar to the morning she found her lifeless mother. Instinctively, she shouts out, "John! John, are you okay?"

She hears a defiant, "I'm fine."

She doesn't believe the words and rushes to lift an almost lifeless body. Suddenly, she understands the meaning of dead weight. Panic-stricken and looking for help, she gasps to herself, "I can't rouse John." She rushes to phone Jay.

6:05 A.M.

"I can't rouse John," a sleepy Joan hears as she picks up the phone beside her bed. Jay's been at the hospital all night with three deliveries. Joan is accustomed to handling family emergencies. She knows Ret is scared.

"Tell Jay," Ret continues.

"We don't need Jay yet. I'm coming right over," Joan replies quickly.

6:45 A.M.

Joan jumps into her car and speeds into Fredericksburg from the Argyle Heights suburbs. As the speedometer hits 70, she remembers to take the new bridge across the Rappahannock River in order to get into town quicker. She is a mass of fears, not the least of which is that the police may stop her. "I'll worry about that later," she convinces herself as her car hurtles across the bridge.

6:50 A.M.

Joan finds the door unlocked, runs up the stairs breathlessly, and races toward the back of the house. She rushes directly into the bedroom, leans over, and takes the pulse. *God, he's out of it,* she thinks. *John's not going to be with us much longer.* Joan hurries to the phone and calls Dave Rice.

"Bring him right to the hospital, and I'll meet you there," the doctor tells her.

Next Joan dials the hospital and reaches Jay. "You'd better get to Retta's right away. I think John is dying."

"Don't call an ambulance yet. I'm on my way."

7:00 A.M.

During the five-minute trip from the hospital, Jay's thoughts wander. *Well, it's obvious what's happened. He's in hepatic coma. I knew John was going to die when I first heard he had varices. It's like the earthquake in California. It is not a question of if, only when. The day he went down in the jungles with all that Buddha stuff, I remember thinking, "You dumb ass, you're grandstanding again and they've got bugs over there that haven't even got names and you ought to stop playing around and get home." I should have brought him back to reality and gotten him home. I should have written him then. Now it's too late.*

7:10 A.M.

Jay arrives and the orderliness of the preparations at the house breaks down. Joan, the Capricorn, takes charge, issues orders. "Retta, call the Rescue Squad."

"No," Jay protests. "That'll take too long. We can get him there ourselves." Retta rushes to the attic and finds an old blanket for a stretcher carry. It doesn't work.

Retta's friend, David, who has just arrived on the scene says, "Stand back. I can carry him down the stairs fireman style."

Joan seems relieved and says, "Lay him gently on the back seat after I pull the car close to the curb."

Retta sits on the floor. Jay jumps in the front, and the group sets off to Mary Washington Hospital, less than a mile away.

7:35 A.M.

At Mary Washington, Bruce Day, an orderly and history buff, is passing the time spinning some Civil War stories with Karen Nunnally. Jay rushes in. The idle chatter stops abruptly when Jay shouts, "I've got somebody outside in hepatic coma. Come quickly."

While Bruce hurries outside, Karen prepares to receive her new patient. After seven years at the Mary Washington Emergency Room, she's seen everything, but still thrives on the excitement and variety that are part of emergency room nursing. Bruce and another orderly return. Karen records, "pulse 90, respirations 20, blood pressure 110/60." After a quick mini-assessment, she writes "code 2" on the admission form. Code 1 is no longer breathing.

Five miles to the north, Janet Payne arrives at Stafford High to begin her teaching day. Sally, the school secretary, tells her, "Retta's brother is in coma."

If he's in coma, he's going to die. I had better be with Retta. She goes directly to the assistant principal and says she will need to have a substitute because of a medical emergency.

7:40 A.M.

David Rice arrives at the Emergency Room, does a quick assessment, and writes initial orders: "blood ammonia, chem 7, take vital signs every half hour." Retta and Joan are in the waiting room, emotionally numb. Everything's been so hectic, Retta has not yet had time to think. She still hasn't grasped the reality of impending death. As she is sitting there collecting herself, a nurse brings her a gold chain and a Medic Alert bracelet. Choking back tears, Retta remarks, "John gave me this

chain before his operation in Bangkok. It's all he has left in the world."
She slips the chain with its Buddha image over her head and keeps it on.

7:46 A.M.

Dr. Rice worries about the destructive nature of the toxins flooding
the system because of the almost total failure of the liver. They must be
removed. He orders a Foley catheter, enemas, neomycin, lactulose, and
an IV drip. He turns to Karen and says, "This is Dr. Robbins' brother.
He has chronic hepatitis B contracted a number of years ago. He has
previously had a portacaval shunt for GI [gastrointestinal] hemorrhaging, and has been fighting encephalopathy [damage to the brain] and
spontaneous peritonitis [an intestinal infection]. He is awaiting a liver
transplant at MCV." Karen's seen people in hepatic coma with the
bloated stomachs and knows they just don't survive. Nevertheless, she
goes to work.

7:50 A.M.

Karen supervises the move to Trauma Room 2. Pulse 90, respirations 80, blood pressure 122/80. She connects the cardiac monitor, calls
for all hospital records, begins the IV of dextrose and water, and places
a Foley catheter. Jay and Joan brood in the waiting room. Jay is
resigned. *He's going to die . . . . I don't remember from med school days
how long it takes for someone in hepatic coma to die. They're not going
to give him a liver at MCV. He's almost 50 and has hepatitis B. They've
been fiddling around now for nine months. Perhaps we should move him
to MCV after all, and let them do an autopsy. We owe them that.*

8:30 A.M.

At the MCV Organ Procurement office in Richmond, Diana Mills
and Christy Heindl are arriving at work.

8:35 A.M.

Trauma Room 2 at Mary Washington: pulse 88, respirations 18,
blood pressure 110/70. Dave Rice walks into the waiting room to report
to Jay, Retta, and Joan. The doctors talk quietly to one another. Jay
whispers to Dave Rice, "I am resolved. I know he will die. Call Dr.
Carithers and see if they want him at MCV or just want to let him die up

here. I don't think he can have a transplant even if they do find a liver. I don't think he can make it to an operation."

Jay returns to Retta and Joan with news that nothing has yet been settled about a move to MCV. They decide to walk across Route 1 and have breakfast at the Hot Shoppes.

9:30 A.M.

The group returns from breakfast, and Retta sees Janet. Retta has her first cry of the day. Time later for tears thinks Capricorn Janet. Lack of organization concerns her. *First, it's really stupid they didn't call the Rescue Squad. Why is John in Fredericksburg and not Richmond? Who's in charge here?*

Retta tells Janet what's happened. "They're preparing to take John to a room at Mary Washington right now."

Janet worries. *Why didn't they take John directly to MCV? He should be at MCV, where they know what they are doing.* She turns to ask Retta if anyone has called Richmond. She hears, "Dr. Rice is going to call."

Joan, the other Capricorn, volunteers, "I think you'd better call Ann Reid." Each Capricorn is eager to take charge, but understands that Retta has always had a special relationship with her younger brother. They defer to her.

9:45 A.M.

Ret decides to use the phone in the Emergency Room lobby to call Ann Reid Priest. She knows the number by heart, because she's learned it during the long wait for a beeper page signaling the availability of a donor liver. She is steady as she punches 1-804-786-0951. "Ann, this is Retta Robbins. John is in hepatic coma. He's in the ER now. I want to notify you. Let us know what we're supposed to do."

Ann Reid replies curtly, "He should be here. I'll take care of it." Ann Reid wastes no more time with Retta. She hangs up and goes to work.

Ann is a combination football quarterback, basketball point guard, and military general. She puts the transplant ball in play and moves the team with all the skill, speed, and precision of a quarterback running a two-minute drill. As the point guard, she must know at all times where and when to feed the ball to the various members of the team. As the general, she must concentrate her troops on the field of battle—the most difficult of all tasks for the commander. Virginia's beloved General Lee failed to concentrate his troops effectively at Gettysburg. It meant the death of the Confederacy. If Ann Reid fails in Richmond this day, her patient will die.

Retta's news hasn't surprised Ann Reid. She is amazed it hasn't happened sooner. She instinctively knows that getting her patient to a place where he can be managed by professionals who know how to deal with hepatic coma is the most important consideration at the moment. MCV's MRICU is that place. Mendez can worry later about the surgery.

9:50 A.M.

Ann Reid calls Bob Carithers. "John Robbins is in coma in Fredericksburg. I have just talked to his sister."

Carithers agrees with Ann's initial reaction to get the patient to Richmond. "Get him here immediately. He needs to be managed by intensivists."

It's Thursday, Carithers' day to be in the clinic. Ann Reid checks with him periodically to let him know how things are going, but manages pretty much on her own until Mendez arrives on the scene to take charge.

Unrelated circumstances complicate Ann's work today and call for all of her skill. She explains to Carithers, "There are no beds available in the ICU." She has to contact Kathy Friedenberg, the unit coordinator for the Medical Respiratory Intensive Care Unit, to see what can be done.

9:53 A.M.

The lack of a free bed in the ICU forces Ann to report to Carithers, "I don't believe we can handle the situation here now."

9:55 A.M.

Dr. Rice calls Dr. Carithers at MCV and says, "John Robbins is here and in coma. He is now stable and needs to come to MCV right away."

Carithers replies, "First, we don't have a prospect of a liver, and we've got a real situation here. I've never seen anything quite like it in my ten years here. There are no ICU beds and in the temporary ICU in the ER, we have a nursing shortage. How is it there?" David Rice—

calm, thorough, and by nature cautious—replies, "We're holding him right now in our ER. We're tight on beds, but we can get him a bed in our Post Surgical Unit. BP 110/60, pulse 88, respirations 16, and it's been in that range since he came to the ER at 7:30. He is semi-comatose. He did swallow some lactulose. We've started a D5W, and his blood sugar is between 40 and 80 mg. We are going to run blood cultures and chemistries and a neomycin enema."

Finally, Carithers broaches the crucial question, "Can you manage him for the day while we intensify the search for a liver?"

"Yes."

"Perhaps then," Carithers concludes, "it is better and safer for him to remain there."

"I agree. We can manage."

10:00 A.M.

Dr. Rice walks into the waiting room and explains the situation. Jay readily agrees with Carithers' and Rice's decision for his brother to remain at Mary Washington for the time being. Joan and Retta stare blankly.

Janet's mad, but swallows her anger. *Damn it! They're just stalling at MCV and are going to let him die here so it won't look bad for them. John doesn't have a chance at all if he doesn't get to MCV.*

Janet wants to blurt out her frustration to Retta and get something done immediately. Her thoughts are like those of almost all transplant families and friends who lose faith and get angry at the doctors and the hospital in the last desperate hours before death. Janet thinks to herself, *MCV is just not going to get John a liver and perform a transplant. They've just been leading everyone on. No bed and a nursing shortage are pretty lame excuses. Month after month we have waited and waited and waited and they never had any serious thought of the transplant. They were just trying to be comforting in the last days. I watched John get weaker and weaker. I've never been around a young person who has died. It just can't happen. I want to tell Retta to do something. They just can't let him die here at Mary Washington. This is absurd.*

In Richmond, both Carithers and Ann Reid understand what is going through a family's mind, but neither ever seriously considers not doing the transplant, even though the coma raises everything several degrees in complexity. The coma means that Mendez will have to try an exceptionally difficult operation under very challenging, emergency conditions. Carithers explains to Ann Reid, "MCV's committed to do the transplant, and we will not back off that commitment just because of the increased difficulty."

Carithers feels that the critical factor in the transplant decision is the condition of the lungs and kidneys. He believes that a transplant would be possible if his patient can be kept stable with no lung problems and if the team can find a liver. Big if's.

Mendez is not as optimistic as Carithers. Ann Reid finds the volatile surgeon as he is making his 10 o'clock rounds at the MRICU.

"Robbins is in coma in Fredericksburg."

That's it, he thinks to himself, *he's done for.* But he replies laconically, "I'll upgrade him to a Status 9 and we'll press the search." Although he is sure that he will never be able to attempt his record-shattering surgery, he does not alter his commitment to the transplant despite the fact that the odds have lengthened considerably.

He explains to the interns, nurses, and others who make up the retinue that follow the surgeon as he parades through the ICU like a potentate receiving tribute from his subjects, "People who have had portacaval shunts die in two ways. First from liver failure and second from falling into a deep, unarousable coma. By now, Robbins has absolutely nothing left. If we find a liver in time, he will enter the OR with no liver reserve whatsoever. In addition, he is slipping closer and closer to an unarousable stage-one coma."

Although the six-month search for the liver did not yield a suitable donor organ, Mendez still has one option left. He turns, walks confidently to the desk area in the center of the ICU that contains the multitude of monitoring equipment, and places a call to Diana Mills at the MCV organ procurement center. "Upgrade Robbins to a Status 9 and make individual calls to all centers within 1500 miles." With that, Mendez goes about his usual Thursday schedule.

Status 9 is reserved for patients in critical condition in the ICU who have fewer than twenty-four hours to live. Status 9 identifies an important distinction, because it speeds the search and enables the team to operate on the basis of possibilities. For example, Diana might charter a plane and Ann Reid could bring the patient to the hospital, assembling the team in hopes that a potential donor's family will give consent. Ordinarily none of these things is done until the family formally signs the documents consenting to organ donation. Today Ann Reid and Diana have no other choice. Time simply will not allow them to follow usual procedures. In these situations they won't get two chances.

Diana turns to computer operator Christy Heindl and says, "Upgrade Robbins to a 9. He's in coma." Christy's watched this name on her computer for six months, read the story in the Richmond *News Leader,* entered the name, and made changes in the file so many times that she thinks of the patient as an old friend. Christy punches in the new data, then she and Diana cross their fingers, make calls, and pray.

It was a much more difficult process than necessary because of the Reagan Administration's opposition to the national computer register for donors and recipients. As a result, quick recovery in emergency situations is little more than luck. Instead of making just one computer entry, Christy and Diane had to begin calling the centers within a 1500-mile range of MCV: Pittsburgh, Norfolk, Durham, Winston-Salem, Nashville, Louisville, Bowling Green, Houston, Dallas, Birmingham, Shreveport, Tampa, Miami, Gainesville, Atlanta, New York, Toronto, and many more.

10:30 A.M.

At MCV, Christy is calling centers throughout the Eastern Seaboard.

In Fredericksburg, Valerie Sherman, the 7-to-3 shift nurse in Mary Washington Hospital's Post Surgical Unit (PSU), looks at the patient she's just received from the ER. Scared when she saw the dry, yellow skin, the recent graduate of nearby Germanna Community College's nursing program has never seen anyone in hepatic coma before. Chuck Rose, a critical care unit coordinator, assigns her this case for experience and stands right beside her.

10:40 A.M.

Dr. Rice arrives at the PSU to make his first assessment, now that he has the patient for at least a day. Jay, Joan, and Retta wait outside the room. Valerie is still settling down in the case. She thinks to herself, *We're going to lose him at any minute or he's going to make medical history. Dr. Robbins' brother is so young, and it's so sad. He's in his forties and that's such a terrible loss.*

10:45 A.M.

Jay, Joan, Retta, and Janet enter the PSU for the first time. Joan tells Jay, "He looks like he is peacefully sleeping. Boy, he looks better."

Jay, however, is not fooled by looks and, with an air of resignation, mutters sadly, "This is what I was afraid of," and he leaves to see his own patients. Retta replaces him and sighs, "He looks peaceful."

11:00 A.M.

Valerie comes into the room to check and take vital signs. Pulse 81, respirations 20, blood pressure 130/70. "He seems stable," she tells Joan, who stands staring at James Monroe High School, visible from the room's windows. She adds, "Talk to him. Try to keep him from going into a deeper coma." Joan crosses her arms and thinks with a sense of resignation, "Jay always said this is the way it would end."

Retta's efforts to rouse her brother lead only to his emitting a few mumbled, nonsensical screams. Discouraged, Retta slips out of the room and, with tears welling up inside her, says quietly to Janet, "You'd better go in now and see John, if . . . ."

She can't finish. Janet understands, hurries into the room, and says, "John, wake up."

And so the time passes in the PSU.

Outside, life bustles. Students come and go across the street at James Monroe High School, and cars pass on busy Route One several hundred yards from the hospital. While one life is ending, other life is going on at its usual pace.

Joan, Janet thinks, is quite prepared for what she believes is going to happen. Janet and Joan talk about Ret, and how she is going to take the death. They fear she might "go off the deep end." Janet is assigned to take care of Ret.

11:30 A.M.

By now the realization of what is happening is dawning more clearly, and Janet gets mad. Janet is a fighter. *This is absurd. Everyone is just standing around waiting for him to die. Something has got to be done. It's just an unfair thing that MCV is not going to give John the transplant after they said they would. If someone with some power did something or said something, the transplant would become a reality. It's just absurd that everybody is just accepting this, and they're just going to let him die right here.*

Joan and Valerie convince Retta that she can leave for a few minutes—that nothing will happen in the amount of time it takes to go home and change her clothes. Janet agrees to take Retta home. Silence fills Janet's Toyota on the trip.

11:50 A.M.

With Retta upstairs changing, Janet paces in frustration. *Something must be done*, she thinks. *But what?* Then suddenly, State Senator Bobby Scott's name jumps into Janet's mind. She runs to the phone and quickly dials his number. Much to her surprise, she hears his voice.

"Bobby Scott." It is the Senator himself.

By coincidence, he happens to be in his office now, a few minutes before noon, in conference with some lobbyists before walking from the General Assembly Building to the Capitol for that day's session of the Senate.

Janet blurts out, "Bobby, you've go to do something. MCV won't talk to us. They won't move him. . . ."

"Now wait a minute Janet," the Senator says, trying to calm her. "Tell me what's happened."

Janet recounts the highlights of the day and finishes with, "First they said they didn't have a bed, then they said they have a nursing shortage. I think they're just lying to us. I don't think they ever intend to transfer him. Somebody has to do something."

"I'll call MCV and get back to you."

It is only minutes before Bobby is supposed to be in his Senate seat. As he leaves his office, he asks legislative aide Joni Ivey to look into the situation. Bobby gets on the elevator, goes down the four floors, out the front door, past the statue of Harry Flood Byrd, and into the Senate chambers.

It's a cold, blustery day in Richmond.

2

...a time to seek,
a time to lose...

It's noon. The drama is six hours old. The cast growing, the stage broadening. Action is taking place in Fredericksburg and Richmond. Telephone calls are being made to locations throughout a 1500-mile radius.

12:15 P.M.

In Fredericksburg, at Mary Washington's PSU, Valerie Sherman repositions her patient and takes vitals: pulse 78, respirations 20, blood pressure 120/70.

12:45 P.M.

In Gainesville, Florida, MCV's "Desperate we have a Status 9" startles one of the workers in the organ procurement office for the Gainesville region. In turn, he calls his contact in the critical care unit at the University of Florida Shands Hospital and learns there may be a potential donor. His heart rate picks up. He suddenly realizes he might have something for MCV. Details are sketchy and, of course, cannot be released, since the patient's confidentiality must be protected. He does, however, learn that the unit has a critically injured young man, nineteen years old, who has been in intensive care since his head trauma injury in an automobile accident three nights ago. Although doctors have not yet initiated procedures for a declaration of brain death, yesterday's EEG was a flat line, one indication of a lack of brain activity.

The Gainesville Organ Procurement Office has no one on the waiting list from the three nearest liver transplant centers: Birmingham, Shreveport, and Durham. That means MCV would get the first chance if something should develop in Gainesville. The procurement official determines to go to Shands and investigate the emerging possibility.

1:00 P.M.

The Virginia Senate has been adjourned now for ten minutes and Joni tells Bobby Scott that Judy Collins is looking into the MCV situation and will call Janet directly. Bobby says good, calls Janet himself, then heads to a meeting of the Senate Transportation Committee.

Bill, the Organ Procurement Officer in Gainesville, calls Diana, his counterpart in Richmond, to report that he is on his way to evaluate a potential donor. Normally Bill would not call a recipient hospital at this stage, but Status 9 changes routine procedures. This liver at Shands may be the MCV patient's only chance in the country. Diana knows that she now has about an hour and half to wait, to see if something develops. She calls Ann Reid, who in turn notifies Mendez and Carithers. Next, Ann Reid talks with the unit coordinator in the ICU about the possibility of moving some patients to make room for the transplant patient.

1:30 P.M.

Bill reaches the critical care unit of the Shands Teaching Hospital in Gainesville and begins his assessment of the potential donor. He does a physical exam, looks at lab reports. He turns to the primary care nurse and asks, "Was he admitted with a hypertensive crisis?" No. Blood pressure levels are within the acceptable range. Weight, size, and blood and tissue types are okay for the MCV patient. Next, he checks the urine output to determine that the kidneys are functioning properly. Finally, he calls for all the laboratory chemistry that is routinely done. In this preliminary examination, Bill looks only at information already a part of the record. He cannot order any special tests.

2:30 P.M.

Nurse Valerie Sherman enters the room in the PSU at Mary Washington Hospital to take vital signs and make neurological checks. Pulse 78, respirations 20, blood pressure 128/70. Questions:

"Who are you?" Silence.

"Where are you?" Silence.

"Who am I?" Silence.

"Squeeze my hand if you understand." No response.

She begins to reposition her patient, who says only, "Oh shit, not this again."

Valerie remarks to Joan, "He's a fighter, isn't he?" She leaves to tell her supervisor, "I'm scared. I have the training, but organ failure is such a different kind of thing. I've never seen a liver like that, and it's frightening because he is such a young person."

2:45 P.M.

Diana and Christy are waiting anxiously in the Organ Procurement Office. Suddenly a ring pierces the silence filling the room. A life hangs in the balance. It's Bill. "So far all the medical criteria are go. He could be a good donor." He gives Diana the pertinent medical information to be relayed to Dr. Mendez. In addition, Bill says the doctors are now beginning a final examination for a declaration of brain death. The information is being gathered and final tests are being made as he and Diana speak. Florida law requires two-flat line EEGs twenty-four hours apart before any declaration of brain death. The final test can't be made until 4 p.m. Then all the data will have to be gathered, with yet another neurologist making the declaration still later. "Are you interested?" Bill asks, in conclusion.

"Yes. I'll contact Dr. Mendez and be right back with you."

Diana puts down the phone, smiles at her colleague Christy, and says, "We've got one working. Robbins may have a shot at it yet." She tracks Mendez down at the McGuire Veterans Center across town and reads him the information on the potential donor: "5'11", 150 pounds, blood type O positive, cardiovascular condition is stable, no previous surgery, no blood transfusions during this hospitalization, no ruptures of the colon or intestines. The donor is a college student and there are no social history red flags. No declaration of brain death and no permission from parents."

The acceptance of the donor organ is, according to Carithers, "a heavy responsibility" for Mendez. In questionable cases, where there are reasonable doubts, he goes to the family of the dying patient and allows the family to participate in the decision. The choice to wait for a better donor, of course, means that the patient might die before a more suitable organ is found. It is only the first in a series of agonizing decisions that doctors and families have to make. In marginal cases, Mendez often calls Carithers to discuss the case.

Carithers explains: "The reasons there are many re-transplants is because often livers don't work. There is a real judgment when to take a liver and when not to take a liver, because the worst thing that can happen in transplant is for the liver not to work." Mendez, Carithers knows, "is very suspicious, very, very conservative. It is not at all unusual for him to turn down a liver, and for Pittsburgh to take it."

Today, Mendez can't be conservative. He will probably have to take anything. "Thank you," Mendez says to Diana. "We're interested." He puts the case on the back burner until brain death is declared and permission is granted. But from this point on he is, in the words of his wife Sharon, in his "liver mode."

3:00 P.M.

In Fredericksburg, Libby Pearson, the 3-to-11 p.m. shift supervisor of nursing at Mary Washington Hospital, begins her shift, checks the charts of critical cases, and learns that Dr. Robbins' brother is in the PSU in hepatic coma.

In Richmond, Mendez's interest sets off a frenzy of almost perpetual motion. Diana calls Ann Reid Priest at MCV to tell her that the recovery team is actively working on a potential liver. Diana puts down the phone and immediately picks it up again to dial the number at Martin Air for Robin Purcell. Robin, who runs the office of the charter air company located at Richmond's Byrd Airport, recognizes Diana's British accent on the phone.

"Robin, we're looking at one. It's real early, don't have a clue, maybe it's 50-50, but what've you got? It's critical and time's short. May be going to Gainesville, so we will want a Lear."

Robin recognizes the feeling building inside her. She knows that Martin Air's Lear 35 is not available, and she will have to find a plane from another charter carrier to make the flight to Gainesville. She starts to work. "Finding the plane," she says, "is such an all-consuming project. Even if you're not actively on the phone, you can't let go of it because it is so critical. You're waiting for somebody to call you back and you feel that you're going to let somebody down—these are not guys going to watch a baseball game in Baltimore. This one counts." For some hours to come, it will not be business as usual for Robin.

She remembers trying to get a plane for a critical patient, a five-year-old boy, when the frustration and responsibility caused her to break out in tears as she sat at her desk. That night she called thirty-five different charter operators. "Everything was ready—the donor, the surgeons, everything. 'Robin, where's the plane?' It's not like taking two drunks to Atlantic City to gamble. With a transplant, we are playing a very significant part in a life-or-death process."

3:15 P.M.

In Gainesville, Bill, from the local organ procurement agency, begins his in-depth physical assessment. He is always "excited" during this phase of the organ recovery and knows he must move quickly but surely, because of the critical nature of the situation. He knows a life is at stake, and every second he saves in the preliminary steps of the process gives the surgeons more time. He moves in to examine the teenage traffic victim. Most organ donors have previously been robust and healthy and, like the young man now lying comatose in the intensive care unit, show no outward signs of the head trauma injury that brings them to their death. Bill knows from long experience that frequently this absence of outward sign of injury makes it so difficult for people to understand brain death.

In Richmond, Ann Reid Priest is setting up her command post at the MRICU on the fourth floor of MCV's main hospital. First she must find a bed. She explains to unit coordinator Kathy Friedenberg, "Although there is as yet no confirmed brain death or donation, once there is confirmation, the donor hospital will want to move quickly. They don't want to waste any time. The bottom line for us is that I've got to move along under several assumptions. I don't have much time, and I don't want to get caught with Robbins not getting to the OR on time. Mendez will go crazy. He'll need all the help and the breaks we can give him. The patient is critical."

Kathy agrees and performs a juggling act by moving a patient to a non-intensive unit and another, less critical patient to a different station in the ICU. Room 513, one of the special rooms for liver transplant patients, is now free. With the room problem solved, Ann Reid puts things in motion to bring her patient from Fredericksburg to Richmond. First, she calls Diana at the procurement office. "Bring in the plane, because we are moving John down from Fredericksburg."

Next she phones Dr. Sally Cook in the MCV Blood Bank. "We're looking at a liver transplant tonight. What's the blood situation? It's Robbins and that's a transplant after a portacaval shunt, so it will be bloody." Cook promises to get right on the situation. She knows it can be tough, because liver transplants are bloody enough anyway. MCV's first liver transplant used a 1000 pints of blood products. She'll check the MCV supply, then if the operation is officially posted with the Operating Room at MCV, call the Richmond Metropolitan Blood Services for more blood supplies.

Ann also knows that because of the critical condition of the patient and the need for speed, the transplant team will have to do something tonight that it has never done before in all its previous transplants: prep a patient for surgery in the MRICU. Usually the team has much more time than tonight's conditions allow. She reviews the staffing situation and asks primary nurse, Chris Wood, "Is someone going to be here or do we have to get another nurse to come in special?" Chris says that Cheryl Wood has just arrived for her 3-to-11 shift and can be assigned exclusively to the new patient. After settling staffing details, Ann Reid calls housekeeping to have a team standing by tonight after pre-op preparations to make sure the room receives the special cleaning and sterilization that only the rooms of liver transplant patients require. Finally, she returns Judy Collins' call to let her know that the patient she is asking about will be moved immediately from Fredericksburg to MCV.

3:30 P.M.

In Fredericksburg, Joan tells Retta to go home, rest, and come back tonight to relieve her. Valerie watches her patient sink and notes, "Pulse 90, respirations 20, blood pressure 110/70, lethargic, repositioned on side, family at bedside."

At Byrd airport, Robin is on the phone to other charter companies. She looks mainly for people she trusts most for their professionalism with crews experienced in this kind of flying. "Jock pilots scare the hell out of the doctors. It is," Robin observes "not a time to bargain-hunt."

3:35 P.M.

Sharon Mendez is at home. She's making an effort for a special meal tonight. It is an unusual day. Her husband is in town and has no surgery. At last a normal evening like a normal couple. The phone rings. She almost doesn't bother to answer because she knows the words by heart: "Baby, we've got a liver going."

She hears the change in his voice as he enters his "liver mode. He's like a different person now, like a performer going on stage."

Not far from the Mendez home, Ray Wallace has finished teaching history at Mils Godwin High School and heads home.

In Fredericksburg, Janet Payne checks her answering machine. "Janet, this is Judy Collins at MCV. You had asked Bobby Scott to check on the situation with John Robbins. The Senator asked me to call you and let you know that preparations are now underway to move Mr. Robbins to MCV." Janet is both relieved and scared. Should she have interfered in what was really a family decision? She wonders, "How am I going to tell Retta?"

3:45 P.M.

Janet is still worrying about telling Retta. She heard Retta come in about five minutes earlier and feels that maybe she should call her. She looks at the phone and, feeling some fear, dials. "Retta, I've done something and I don't know if you're going to be angry or not." She relates the Bobby Scott-Joni Ivey-Judy Collins adventure.

Retta responds without emotion. "Well, I don't know what's going to happen. Do you think they are going to transfer him?"

"That's what she told me they were going to do."

Retta isn't sure. She knows Bobby has influence, and Janet thinks he can do anything. But this? "No way." She dismisses Janet's news and tries to relax for a few minutes. By this time, Ann Reid is in the final stages of orchestrating the move to Richmond. She reaches for the phone to call the 3-to-11 nursing supervisor at Mary Washington. Libby Pearson is just about to leave the nursing office when the phone rings. Ann Reid explains, "I think we may have liver, and we've got to make plans to move Mr. Robbins as soon as possible. We'll send an ambulance for him."

"I don't think that's necessary. I believe we have transportation available right here at the hospital. Let me check on it," Libby says.

"Okay, then. I've got other things to arrange, but I'll be back to you within the hour."

Robin, too, is on the phone. She's talking with Ken Malcomson of Executive Air in Salisbury, Maryland, two hundred miles from Richmond. "We need a Lear for a liver flight to Gainesville. What's available?"

"Our Lear's out on a flight now and won't be available until tomorrow. Sorry."

4:00 P.M.

Libby Pearson contacts the transportation office at Mary Washington. Technician Beverly Payne and driver Keith Jones are getting ready to leave for the day. "Stay put," Libby cautions. "I think we will have a critical patient to send to MCV for a liver transplant."

Three stories above, Valerie Sherman glides quietly into the room and whispers to Joan, "There's a call from MCV for anyone in the family." Joan hurries to the phone at the command desk of the PSU and hears the calm voice of the general, Ann Reid, "We're moving John to Richmond. We think we've found a liver."

Sinking to the floor, Joan gasps, "My God, they are going to try and save him! I didn't think there was any hope of getting a liver in time. My God, he's got a chance!" Always planning, Joan asks Libby Pearson, "Do we have to arrange for an ambulance?"

"No," Libby responds. "The hospital has an ambulance to transport patients."

Thank God. The Auxiliary was right in raising money to buy that ambulance for the hospital, Joan thinks, remembering her activity in that organization.

4:05 P.M.

Joan rushes to the bedside. "John, they've found you a liver." No response. "John, they have found you a liver. This is what you have been waiting for, and it's going to happen. They're going to move you to Richmond. If you understand me, squeeze my hand." No response whatsoever. Looking for any good sign, Joan points to the heart monitor and says to the nurse. "Look! His heartbeat changed!"

Retta is at home, unaware of what just happened at Mary Washington. She thinks, *Perhaps I should call Ray to let his friends know. John was so appreciative of their help, and he made a list of people he wanted to notify. I can't find the list, but Ray will know everyone.*

Sadness, frustration, tears, curses, and anger flow freely. Ret begins, "Ray, this is Ret."

"Hey Ret, how we doing?"

She's distraught. Ray's scared, thinks, *John's dead.* Tears flow.

"John's in irreversible coma at Mary Washington, Ray."

They vent the frustration and anger typical of transplant patients' family and friends in these circumstances.

"Why did the hospital let him get so sick?"

"They never had any intention of transplanting."

"Those bastards never had any intention of finding him a liver."

"They just led us on."

"Goddamn sons of bitches."

"Lying bastards!"

Ray concludes, "Ret, please keep me informed. I'll pass the word on to John's friends here in Richmond and at Hampden-Sydney."

In Fredericksburg, pretty sure the transfer will be soon, Libby Pearson is preparing charts, filling out forms, and making copies of the reams of necessary paperwork. Joan is looking for Jay. He is nowhere to be found and isn't answering the phone at home. Libby thinks the most difficult task at this hour is locating Jay.

4:10 P.M.

Ray is phoning the network. He calls classmate Lewis Drew. Lew is still at a meeting, but Ray talks to Nell, who drawls gently, "Ray, you and Lewis and Billy have done all you possibly could."

"Yes, I guess we have," Ray replies grimly.

4:15 P.M.

Retta is still trying to relax when the phone rings. "Retta," Joan, speaking in an excited tone, says, "They're going to move John. They've found a liver."

Retta catches her breath and manages a hurried, "I'm on my way." She hangs up and races to the hospital.

At MCV, Diana notifies Robin to bring a plane to Richmond as soon as she locates one.

4:20 P.M.

Before rushing out of the house, Retta makes a brief, breathless call to Janet. "They're moving John to Richmond. They're getting a liver for him."

Janet is overwhelmed; her mind races. *I knew Bobby Scott was powerful, but this is just too much. What could he have done that suddenly all of this is happening?*

Richard Xiffo of U.S. Jet Charter in Washington calls Robin at Hawthorne Aviation in Richmond and confirms that they have a Lear 35 available. Xiffo now begins the process of assembling a crew. He must call in Capt. Ed Moston and First Officer Sam Eltonhead and begin the preparations for launch. Moston and Eltonhead leave their homes in nearby areas of Northern Virginia and begin the drive to Washington's National Airport, home base for U.S. Jet. Xiffo calls Robin and says they can be ready to launch around 6 p.m.

4:35 P.M.

Robin calls Diana in the MCV organ procurement office and says the plane can be ready by 6 p.m. "Okay, bring it right now. We don't have the luxury of time to wait for brain death and consent before getting the plane here."

"Okay, they'll be coming from Washington and should be here at 7 p.m."

"Fine, we'll be there, lovely, thank you."

Robin hopes everything goes according to schedule tonight because frequently it does not. Often the flight coordinator says, "Fine, we can be there. Let us gather the crew, throw on some fuel, and we'll be there." But all kinds of unforeseen problems can happen. The flight coordinator can't find the pilot; he's stuck in the terrible traffic of Washington or playing golf. Or the regular co-pilot suddenly decided to get married. Or they found water in the gas in the regular fuel truck and they need to bring in another truck. Or the pilot's seat microphone isn't working for some reason. Or the plane's radar is out. It could be almost anything.

Meantime, the surgeons are waiting. That tends to produce unhappy surgeons. When surgeons are unhappy, everyone in the area becomes unhappy. A late flight throws off the whole schedule all down the line and affects OR time. Time spent waiting for planes is operating room time lost. In transplant, OR time is as scarce as a quiet surgeon.

Next, Robin races over to the local seafood shop and buys a five-pound bag of colossal shrimp and all the trimmings to make a shrimp tray for the surgeons. "They love it; it's their favorite."

4:45 P.M.

The phone rings in Libby Pearson's office. Ann Reid, sounding urgent, says, "Bring Mr. Robbins down. We want him now, as soon as you can get him here."

"Air or ground?"

"The liver is not even in Richmond yet. Ground will be fine. You do have transportation, don't you?"

"Yes. He should be out of here by 6 P.M. and in Richmond by seven."

Libby must find a nurse specialist to accompany technician Beverly Payne and driver Keith Jones in the ambulance. Because of the patient's critical condition, Libby has to find a specially qualified nurse to accompany Beverly. Marsha McGaffic, who has previously accompanied a critically ill young Swedish exchange student on his way to MCV for a heart transplant, happens to be on duty. She is a certified critical care nurse and holds an advanced life support certificate as well. Fortunately, Libby can adjust the schedule and allow her to make the trip. She does not have to wait to call in another nurse. Precious time is saved.

5:15 P.M.

Ray Wallace, as is his usual habit in the late afternoon, is listening to National Public Radio's "All Things Considered." The phone rings. He reaches over and turns down the radio.

"Ray, this is Retta. You're not going to believe this. I'm at the hospital. They're packing John up, and we are on our way to MCV."

Retta tells Ray the story as she understands it. Ray, happy but far from mollified, feels, "Those bastards had the liver all the time, Retta."

"I think you're exactly right, Ray." A little more MCV bashing follows, and Retta confesses, "Jay thinks this is all for naught."

Marsha McGaffic gets her first look at the charts that indicate her patient is rapidly becoming worse. She is apprehensive about the impending trip.

Robin calls Diana to say she is staying on at Hawthorne. Diana assures her that all systems are go, and they are awaiting final word of brain death and consent. The patient should be at MCV around 7 p.m. Diana next calls the MCV surgeons. Dr. Marc Posner will make the trip to Gainesville and do the harvest. Mendez stays in Richmond to open the patient and sew in the new liver.

5:20 P.M.

Ray is alerting the Hampden-Sydney network. Again he reaches Nellie. "This is it, isn't it?" she says. Ray next calls Bill Ware. "I'm just incredulous that this is all happening now when we had just about given up all hope. I'll call John's Theta Chi fraternity brothers," Ware promises Ray.

5:30 P.M.

The neurologists in Gainesville have collected all the evidence, and their report is now ready for the primary care doctor. The reports reads: "no response to external stimuli, no reflex activity, no pupillary response to light, no corneal reflex, no eye movement with caloric testing, no gag reflex, and no cough reflex. The second EEG in a twenty-four hour period is still a flat line, cerebral angiography and radio nuclide brain scan show absence of blood flow to the brain." All requirements of Florida law have been met, and the doctors' conclusion is unequivocal: the nineteen-year-old college freshman is brain dead.

The doctor must now tell the young man's parents. He hates this part of his job. He asks Bill from the Organ Procurement Office, to come with him and wait outside the family room in case the parents want to talk to him. As they walk down the corridor of the hospital, Bill confesses to the doctor, "This is so hard, watching them feel this kind of pain. I once thought I'd get accustomed to it, but I don't think I ever will." He pauses, then adds, "I don't think I want to get accustomed to it." The doctor nods in agreement.

First, the doctor tells the teenager's parents that their son has suffered brain death. He takes time to express his sorrow to the parents, telling them he recognizes the terrible pain they are feeling as they confront the tragic death of their son. But even as he speaks, he can't forget that time is critical now, that he needs to move forward quickly. All those involved in the retrieval of an organ—doctors, officials of the procurement agency—are aware that they might appear insensitive, but they are desperately weighing their need to hurry against the family's grief. It's not easy for anyone. It's a difficult tightrope to walk.

The doctor continues. "I am so sorry. We did all that is humanely possibly."

"What must we do now?" asks a grieving mother.

"You have three options and we do not wish to rush your decision, but it is part of my job to make you aware of them now. Please take your time and think them over. First, you can leave your son on life-support and wait for his organs to wear out. Second, you can execute the natural death act and take him off the ventilator. Or third, you may wish to consider organ donation. If you wish to consider organ donation, I will ask an official from the organization that arranges donations to come in and speak with you. He, I believe, will be able to answer your questions better than I if this is the option you choose."

Several family members respond almost simultaneously, "We'd like to hear more about donation."

The family, in the midst of its grief, is still able to think of another human being. This makes transplant such an incredible phenomenon, as, in the midst of grief, a mother and father are able to think of relieving another family's pain.

The doctor leaves to ask Bill to come back with him and speak to the family. Bill enters the scene and approaches the parents respectfully. The room is filled with questions:

How will the organ be retrieved?

Will it delay the funeral?

Will doctors or medical students perform the surgery?

Will there be any cost?

Can we have an open-casket funeral?

How soon must we decide?

An agony of decision faces a grief-stricken family.

Bill answers the questions as carefully and compassionately as he can. There is no attempt to convince the family to donate. Respecting the family's grief and privacy, he concludes. "Please talk this over privately and if you want any more information, I will be in the unit. Just ask a nurse for me and I will be available at your convenience."

The doctor concludes, "Once again, I am very sorry. Please let us know when you have made your decision."

In Fredericksburg, Marsha McGaffic sees her patient for the first time. "Hello," she says quietly to Joan. "My name is Marsha McGaffic, and I will be going to Richmond in the ambulance with your brother-in-law."

"Should one of us ride with you?" Joan asks.

"No, that's not necessary." In fact, Marsha hopes someone in the family will not insist on being in the ambulance. That, she knows, is never good. She will have her hands full with the patient, and if an emergency develops, she does not want to devote any of her energy and time to caring for a hysterical family member. Joan and Retta understand.

In Richmond, Pat Bezak comes out the front door of Richmond Metropolitan Blood Services, where she has finished her work as Manager of Donor and Hospital Resources. She says goodbye to Medical Director Russell Briere, walks to her car, pulls out into Westwood Avenue, and begins her trip across the James River to her home in Chesterfield County.

5:35 P.M.

Diana calls Ann Reid at MCV and says that brain death has been declared. They are now awaiting parental consent. She has already called Robin, who is now on the phone to U.S. Jet in Washington. "Are you sure of your schedule? Please launch as soon as possible." She puts down the phone and continues work on her shrimp tray.

5:45 P.M.

Beverly Payne and Keith Jones leave the transport office at Mary Washington Hospital, drive the ambulance to the ER dock, and go to the third floor to help the nurses with the transfer. They introduce themselves to Retta and Joan.

At Washington's National Airport, Capt. Ed Moston and First Officer Sam Eltonhead arrive to make final preparations for the charter flight. They know this is a transplant flight, so everything moves at a quicker pace. Eltonhead files the flight plan on the Lifeguard System, identifying the flight as a medical emergency, giving it first priority for takeoff and landing. They'll need that in the busy, early evening rush at National. Moston is busy making preflight preparations. Eltonhead checks the weather. They're lucky. No snow. Last week's major winter storm closed the Richmond airport, but tonight the weather looks good all the way to Gainesville, and it should hold until their return sometime in the early hours of the following morning.

In Fredericksburg, David has been sent by Retta to wake Jay, since he has not responded to the phone. Upon being gently shaken awake, Jay squints at the window, sees the dusk of a February evening outside, and mistakes it for morning.

"Go fix yourself a cup of coffee and some cereal, and I'll be right with you," he tells David.

6:00 P.M.

In Gainesville, it's decision time.

"How can he be dead?" A father asks in frustration and disbelief. "There is not a mark on his beautiful body. He is so young, with the whole world in front of him. He's a college student with a wonderful future. I just don't know." A mother's response comes quickly and surely, "Yes, I want to donate. He heard a program on donation at school, thought it was a wonderful idea . . . signed a donor card . . . talked to me about it."

Slowly the talk turns to the excitement of life, to how a tragedy can result in the saving of many lives. The parents discuss the various aspects of the painful need to decide. Finally, the decision is made. Papers are signed, giving at least four persons a chance to live. Some of the gloom of the three days since the accident is, for the time being, erased.

3

...a time to weep,
a time to laugh...

It's six p.m. and the drama is now twelve hours old. The cast of characters and the area of action are both steadily increasing. Far to the south in Gainesville, parents sign the formal papers donating their son's heart, liver, and kidneys. He lies brain dead not far away in the intensive care unit. Bill from the local organ procurement agency, after calling his counterpart in Richmond, moves into the room to take charge of managing the donor until the organs can be retrieved by the surgeons who will arrive from Richmond and Birmingham. He must keep the brain-dead teenager's blood circulating in his lifeless body long enough for the surgeons to harvest the organs.

In Fredericksburg, the transport team lifts its comatose charge to a gurney for the trip downstairs to the waiting ambulance. Nurses Marsha McGaffic, Beverly Gonzales, and Libby Pearson, along with technician Beverly Payne and ambulance driver Keith Jones, are handling the move. Retta and Joan are watching the proceedings with both terror and the first glimmer of hope they have allowed themselves in twelve hours. Jay is at last awake, preparing to head to Mary Washington.

In Washington, pilots Sam Eltonhead and Ed Moston are preparing their Lear 35 for the flight to Richmond to pick up the MCV team and then on to Gainesville to retrieve the liver.

Preparations are in high gear at many locations throughout Richmond. At Byrd Airport, Robin Purcell from the air charter company is preparing for the arrival of the plane from Washington and the surgeons from downtown Richmond. She is working on her shrimp tray. Diana Mills and Christy Heindl are in the organ procurement office. At MCV, Ann Reid Priest is in her command post at the MRICU, coordinating the efforts of a growing number of health-care professionals. Dr. Carithers is finishing clinic hours and preparing to go home. Dr. Mendez is in his office at the Nelson Clinic, staring at the bumper sticker stuck to his wall, "Don't Bury Kidneys, Transplant Them." Marc Posner, the transplant surgeon who will harvest the donor liver, and his intern assistant, John Alspaugh, are putting on their scrubs in the ER area of MCV, waiting for Diana to pick them up to go to the airport for the flight to Gainesville. Nurses Barbara Parish and Debbie Grant are on duty in the operating room area of MCV. Critical care nurse Cheryl Wood is in the MRICU, preparing to receive her new patient. Jane Evanchyk arrives at her desk in the operating area of MCV, getting ready to begin her duties as charge nurse on the OR floor.

In many locations throughout the Richmond area, others are playing or preparing to play active roles in the growing transplant drama. Ray Wallace is at home calling friends. Pat Bezak from Richmond Metropolitan Blood Services has just picked up her nine-year-old daughter, Yvonne, at the Small World Nursery in Chesterfield County. Blood Services Director Russell Briere is getting ready for dinner with his wife at their condominium, The Warsaw, in the Fan District of Richmond. John Beeston, Sandy Witherington, Ty Aaron, and Janice Rossi, all members of the transplant team, are at their homes, which are scattered throughout the Richmond suburbs.

Slowly but steadily, Ann Reid is concentrating her troops on the battlefield of the operating room. Tonight's is a particularly tricky maneuver because she usually has more time. Nurses, anesthesiologists, perfusionists, and blood supplies all have to be assembled. And it all has to be done to conform to Dr. Mendez's schedule. It's going to be a long night.

6:05 P.M.

Ann Reid Priest is busy. She calls Sally Cook at the blood bank to notify Richmond Blood Services that MCV will be doing a liver transplant tonight and that blood will be necessary. Next, she goes into the intensive care unit to find Cheryl Wood and supervises her preparation to receive the patient who is on his way from Fredericksburg. Mendez, acting much like the director of a space mission, is figuring out the time schedule he wants everyone to follow. "What time do they want us in Gainesville?" Mendez asks Ann Reid.

"Nine p.m."

First, Mendez calculates the time the supporting cast will need. The plane reaches Gainesville by 9 p.m. It will take two hours for Posner and his staff to harvest the liver and another hour to pack it, get it ready, and return to the plane. Flying time is about an hour and half. The liver should be back in Richmond by 2 a.m. He adds one hour for delays and mistakes. Next, Mendez calculates operating room time in Richmond. He allows an hour and a half for the anesthesiologists to get the patient ready, two hours to take out the diseased liver, and adds an hour to that because the portacaval shunt makes additional surgery in the area more time-consuming as well as riskier. Next, the surgeon announces, in the ex cathedra manner of a pope, "I want Robbins in the operating room at 9 p.m."

The schedule now set, everything focuses on following Mendez's timetable. If all works according to plan, the new liver should be going in around 3 a.m. Finally, he lists the pre-op medications then goes to the doctors' lounge to brood and get ready for the biggest technical challenge of his career.

In Washington, Capt. Ed Moston and First Officer Sam Eltonhead proceed to their plane. Henceforth, they are known as Lifeguard 45 Charlie Poppa.

In Gainesville, parents say their final goodbyes to a son. After they leave the ICU, Bill, as the representative of the organ retrieval service, moves in to begin the tricky task of managing the donor. Although he has already been declared brain dead, the teenager's blood, necessary to preserve the vital organs, must still circulate through his body. If the artificial ventilator does not keep him breathing until harvest, or if the body simply wears out to the extent that it can't respond to the life-support machine, the organs will be of no use to the transplant surgeons. If this happens, the MCV patient dies because, in his condition, he won't get a second chance.

First, Bill compiles a detailed medical history. He gives the parents a list of things that may preclude organ donation and asks, "Do you know of anything that would prevent your son from being a good donor?" He examines the medical records to look for history of chronic renal impairment and to assure himself that the donor is free from transmissible disease and malignancy. He goes over all the blood cultures that have already been taken and orders tests for venereal disease, the AIDS virus, hepatitis B, and liver function. He continues to monitor cardiac enzyme tests and serum creatinine and blood urea nitrogen levels. Bill is going to be very busy until the recovery teams arrive. All information must be ready and complete. If it isn't, he will bear the wrath of Marc Posner.

Until the heart is removed and the machines are turned off, the organ procurement officer is in charge of maintaining the donor. He must watch for sixty separate functions, from cardiac output and fluid volume deficiencies to a potential for infection. He no longer calls MCV unless the patient stops breathing, which is possible even while he is on the ventilator.

6:10 P.M.

Jane Evanchyk, the coordinator of the MCV operating suite, is busy making preparations for the surgery. Even though transplants have become routine at MCV, a feeling pervades the operating suite that something special is going on. Everyone moves with a heightened sense of urgency. Jane posts the operation for OR 15, one of the three transplant rooms; sends to the pharmacy for drugs; calls Sandy Witherington and Ty Aaron, the perfusionists, and Janice Rossi, the circulating nurse, to report to the operating suite. Finally, she notifies anesthesiology.

In Fredericksburg, nurse Marsha McGaffic disconnects the IV from her patient, connects the cardiac monitors, transfers him to the gurney, and begins the trip to the waiting ambulance. Retta and Joan watch with a mixture of horror, apprehension, and hope.

6:15 P.M.

Diana Mills leaves the organ procurement office in the Sheltering Arms Building at the MCV complex and goes to the parking deck to get the transplant car, a siren-and-flashing-light equipped Chevrolet donated to the transplant program by Martin Chevrolet of Richmond. John Beeston, the nurse anesthetist, leaves his home, walks to his Thunderbird, and begins his trip to the hospital. He will use the Powhite Freeway and Interstate 95 to reach MCV in about a half-hour.

Beverly and Marsha place their patient in the ambulance, tie down the IV pumps, connect the oxygen, put the monitor above the bed where it can be seen easily, and begin taking vitals. Beverly makes the first entry in her log of the trip. "Mr. Robbins is in a near comatose state. He does not follow commands, but will react to loud verbal stimuli . . . does [not] show any obvious cardiac or respiratory distress. EKG shows normal size rhythm. The right IV is without redness or swelling with D5W pump at 100 ml/hr. Foley catheter is in place." Keith Jones turns the key, the motor roars on, and the ambulance pulls away from the ER dock.

Fifty miles to the north, at National Airport, Capt. Ed Moston speaks to the tower. "Tower, this is Lifeguard 45 Charlie Poppa. Request taxi instructions."

"Roger, Lifeguard 45 Charlie Poppa, taxi to runway one five."

Fifty miles to the south, Mills yells to Posner and Alspaugh, "Let's go." The three members of the recovery team, already dressed in scrubs, take their places in the transport car as it leaves the ER entrance at MCV and heads to nearby Interstate 64 for the rendezvous with Moston and Eltonhead at Byrd Field.

The jets roar on. The Lear backs out of its blocks. An ambulance, a car, a plane, and eight people are now in motion with but one object: to deliver a patient and a liver to the MCV operating room in time to save a life.

6:30 P.M.

Pat Bezak is at home in Richmond. She has just settled in her young daughter from day care and is preparing supper. The phone disturbs her routine. Sally Kirk from the inventory department at Richmond Blood Services asks, "MCV has a liver transplant tonight. Can we support it?"

"I think we can," Pat replies, "but I must check with Dr. Briere." She's happy that Briere is not out of town at his farm today. It's Thursday and he'll be here in Richmond getting ready for dinner with his wife. Pat knows the blood supply is pretty good, and this probably won't be a difficult call. She shudders each time she makes the call, though, as she remembers the time she and Briere could not give permission for a transplant because of a low blood supply, and a critical patient died before another liver could be found.

6:35 P.M.

Passing along fast-food alleys that line entrances to interstates, Jay remarks to Retta and Joan, "You all never got me the pizza you promised last night."

Joan replies a little testily, "Jay, it still is last night!"

And he's driving the car! Retta thinks.

So goes the trip to Richmond. No one talks about the pending operation.

6:37 P.M.

58 AB positive red blood cells, 60 random platelets, 60 A positive blood plasma, 20 A positive corryl units—only seven minutes after the initial request, the first blood shipment for the transplant cranks out of the blood service's computer and is on its way downtown to MCV.

Mendez is in the doctors' lounge area on the fifth-floor operating suite at MCV's main hospital. All flamboyance is gone. Mendez is getting ready. He has planned this operation over and over. This will be his ultimate technical challenge. He plans no new techniques, though the man who invented the operation, Thomas Starzl of the University of Pittsburgh, says it can't be done on someone who has had a portacaval shunt. Tonight, Mendez is on the verge of defying that admonition. His emotions, like those of an athlete before the big game, have been building all day. He reviews his plan and considers all the contingencies. He's done the whole operation in his mind four or five times already: *Are we going to be able to take the shunt down? Clamp above or below the shunt? If one maneuver doesn't work, what's the fallback?*

Over and over he examines the operation in his mind trying to figure out every conceivable move. He doesn't want any surprises that could be avoided by careful planning. There will be surprises enough anyway. He knows the key to liver transplant surgery is a careful plan and an ability to react quickly to changing circumstances. Brain surgeons are careful, methodical plodders. Liver transplant surgeons are the classy, think-on-your-feet, react-to-the-curve-ball, flashy, bombastic trial lawyers of medicine. Mendez can't wait to get in the operating room. This is his big one. For Mendez, tonight is the All-Star game, the seventh game of the World Series, and the Super Bowl all rolled into one. He has felt the excitement building all day. He is reflective and, for an uncharacteristic moment, quiet. He's psyching himself up for the challenge ahead. He has a kind of double emotion. "There's a great responsibility of a life—a new life—in my hands, but at the same time there's an excitement of a technical challenge."

6:39 P.M.

The ambulance is speeding, with sirens blaring, through the dark of a February night. Out of Fredericksburg, through Spotsylvania County and into Caroline County. The signs read like a history book: Spotsylvania Battlefield; the Matta, Po, and Ni rivers; Jackson's Shrine.

Beverly Payne notes, "pulse 88, respirations 20, blood pressure 104/70," and asks, "Are you still with us, John?" Beverly and Marsha continue to shout in an effort to elicit some response. "We don't want him to get into a deeper coma," Marsha remarks to Beverly. "Gosh, his color is so awful—yellow and jaundiced."

Mendez is preparing himself. *I'm not being paid to be second or third. I'm being paid to be the best. I'm not going into that operating room to say, 'Let's try it, let's see what happens.' I'm there because I'm supposed to be the best there is. And, if not, I'm supposed to be striving to be the best there is.*

6:40 P.M.

"Tower, this is Lifeguard 45 Charlie Poppa, ready for takeoff, runway one five."

"Roger, Lifeguard 45 Charlie Poppa, cleared for takeoff."

6:42 P.M.

"Departure, this is Lifeguard 45 Charlie Poppa. I'm at a thousand feet."

"Roger, cleared to climb to nine thousand, turn left to heading two zero zero."

6:53 P.M.

Marsha McGaffic leans over her patient. "Are you still with us, John?"

"Yes."

They are pleased. Beverly says excitedly, "Look, he's fighting. He doesn't know what's happening. He's just fighting. Some people don't fight. They give up and do nothing at all. This is a good sign. Maybe we're going to get him there after all."

6:55 P.M.

"Richmond approach, this is Lifeguard 45 Charlie Poppa at nine thousand. Request landing instructions."

The transplant car with Mills, Posner, and Alspaugh has passed the passenger terminal. It continues by the sign that reads "Dead End" and pulls up at Hawthorne Aviation.

In the ambulance, Marsha turns to Beverly and says, "He's right on the edge of being totally comatose. He's going to be totally comatose by dawn. He's sinking quickly. Where are we, Keith?"

"Approaching the Belevidere toll plaza. I'll call MCV when we pass that marker."

7:00 P.M.

The Mary Washington ambulance passes the first toll plaza on the Richmond-Petersburg Turnpike. Keith Jones reaches for his HEAR radio, punches the code for MCV, and says, "We're about five minutes away. Patient unstable." He hears, "Go to the Medical ER dock, and everyone will be waiting."

At MCV, Barbara Parish, a circulating nurse for the OR, has arrived and is beginning to stock the operating room for the night's transplant. John Beeston is also there preparing the anesthetists' equipment. Sandy Witherington and Ty Aaron have arrived from home and are beginning to set up the perfusion machine. The nurses usually get a headache during this tense time because there is so much to do to prepare for such a long operation. They know they will be working with a battery of surgeons who themselves are under extreme pressure and often take it out on everyone else in the OR. All this combines to produce a period of unpleasant apprehension and tension. As they are working, Beeston tells Parish, "This is the guy who was a professor, who went abroad and got hepatitis."

Christy Heindl has already arrived on the scene from the procurement offices. She plugs in the red transplant phone and establishes her command post for the operation. She will be the communications officer between Diana Mills in Gainesville with the recovery team and Nurse Barbara Parish with the transplant team in Richmond. Christy's phone rings. Diana tells her that the recovery team is at the airport and about to board the plane. She relays the first ETA for Gainesville.

7:01 P.M.

"Richmond tower, this is Lifeguard 45 Charlie Poppa. Request final landing instructions."

7:05 P.M.

Moston guides the Lear to the landing area at Hawthorne Aviation, cuts one engine, and prepares to receive the recovery team on board.

7:10 P.M.

"Tower, this is Lifeguard 45 Charlie Poppa. Request taxi instructions." Doctors Posner and Alspaugh and nurse Diane Mills are in the rear of the plane, belts tightened. Posner, a white-knuckle flier, is always nervous about takeoffs. He winces and tolerates this unpleasant aspect of the challenge of transplant surgery.

"Roger, Lifeguard 45 Charlie Poppa. Taxi to runway two zero."

In downtown Richmond, the Mary Washington ambulance rolls up the street, turns left behind the White House of the Confederacy, and comes to a halt at the ER entrance. Marsha, Beverly, and Keith unload their patient quickly and rush by the ER doctors, who wave them through to the intensive care units.

"Clearance Delivery, this is Lifeguard 45 Charlie Poppa, to Gainesville." Eltonhead makes notes of route, altitude, and other navigational details for the flight to the Florida city.

7:15 P.M.

Marsha McGaffic turns her patient over to the nurses at the MRICU and is immediately impressed by the MCV operation. A well-oiled, experienced, and disciplined team swings into high gear. Nurse Cheryl Wood receives her patient and begins pre-op medications within the first two minutes of arrival. Dozens of nurses, lab technicians, interns, residents, and attending physicians join her.

In Gainesville, Bill is concerned about an impaired gas exchange in the donor's condition. He moves to monitor the mechanical ventilator more carefully, obtains some arterial blood gas readings, and repositions the teenager to administer chest physiotherapy. He's got to maintain his patient's ability to supply blood to the essential organs.

"Tower, this is Lifeguard 45 Charlie Poppa, ready for takeoff, runway two zero."

"Roger, Lifeguard 45 Charlie Poppa, cleared for takeoff."

Marc Posner doesn't like to fly on "those little planes." He says he is always, "a little anxious until I have the liver in my hands and am on the way back, because anything can happen. I don't feel comfortable until I have the liver in my hands. I just have this feeling—it's not a terrible overwhelming feeling. It's just a little bit of anxiety."

7:17 P.M.

"Departure, this is Lifeguard 45 Charlie Poppa, I'm at a thousand feet."

"Roger, Lifeguard 45 Charlie Poppa, cleared to climb to nine thousand, turn left to heading two two zero."

7:30 P.M.

The MRICU intern, Greg Loundrey, logs the new patient's arrival at MCV in what will be the first of thousands of entries in the progress reports. "Patient is a 47-year-old white male with liver failure due to chronic active hepatitis. Admitted for liver transplant."

7:35 P.M.

"Lifeguard 45 Charlie Poppa, this is Washington Center. Contact Atlanta Center on frequency 133.2."

"Roger, Washington Center, Lifeguard 45 Charlie Poppa contacting Washington Center on 133.2."

Nurse Wood injects the first dose of the antibiotic inpenum, which is to be given over the next twelve hours. She confirms that twenty units each of packed cells, fresh frozen plasma and platelets have already arrived.

7:40 P.M.

Retta, Jay, and Joan arrive at the MRICU and are met by Ann Reid, who escorts them to a small room near the entrance to the unit.

The recovery team, currently 39,000 feet above the low flatlands of the coastal Carolinas, is well on its way to Gainesville. They are still about an hour from the Florida city, home to the University of Florida. The route will keep the Lear close to the coast until it reaches Jacksonville, before it heads inland for Gainesville. Diana calls the organ procurement coordinators in Richmond and at Shands Hospital in Gainesville with the expected time of arrival.

In the plane, Posner is relaxing. The weather's not too bad, and it looks like they will make the trip okay weatherwise. Posner is a thirty-eight-year-old surgeon and number-one assistant to Mendez. He got into medicine and transplant surgery in a roundabout way. A Phi Beta Kappa undergraduate philosophy major at Bucknell University, he was all ready to go to Columbia to pursue a Ph.D. when suddenly he realized that he was burned out on philosophy, and he searched around for something else. A good child of the sixties, he had been a member of the SDS and opposed the Vietnam War. A high lottery number allowed him the luxury of taking a year off to think. He ended up living in a commune and picking artichokes in Salinas, California. He ultimately found his way to surgery and transplants by way of medical school and internship.

Posner is a worrier, and tonight's case troubles him more than usual. He knows that people in coma before liver transplant have only a twenty-five percent chance of survival. In tonight's case those odds are even slimmer because of the portacaval shunt. He wonders, *Is Mendez going to be able to take that shunt down? Is Robbins ever going to come out of coma? I wonder why Mendez took that case? Boy, coma is such a bad way to start out.*

He knew many liver transplant centers would not even make the attempt—Mayo Clinic just doesn't transplant patients with long odds. Mendez is going up against high odds. It's going to be a long night.

8:00 P.M.

Ann Reid and Greg Loundrey, the intensive care unit intern, join Retta, Jay, and Joan in the small room where they've been waiting. Loundrey gives Jay the consent form for the transplant and begins an explanation. Jay interrupts. "Look, give me a break. I'm a doctor. I know what's up. It's the only chance he's got." He signs for his comatose brother. While Retta is calmed by the team's efficiency, Jay still has doubts. He hasn't see the donor liver yet.

"Lifeguard 45 Charlie Poppa, this is Atlanta Center. Contact Jacksonville Center on frequency 162.2." The plane, above the Georgia coast, is approaching north Florida, preparing to head inland to Gainesville.

8:15 P.M.

Retta, Jay, and Joan gather in the last minutes before surgery. Retta talks constantly, trying to reassure herself. "John, you look wonderful. You are going to have a new liver. They are going to give you something, and you are going feel all right. Everything is just the way they planned."

8:20 P.M.

High in the sky above the Florida panhandle, the plane with the organ recovery team begins its descent to nine thousand feet in preparation for landing.

8:42 P.M.

"Gainesville Approach, this is Lifeguard 45 Charlie Poppa at nine thousand. Request landing approach."

In Richmond, Janet Payne is awed by what she sees unfolding before her eyes. *It's like being in a movie,* she thinks. *The action and tension are mounting. This is dramatic and John's doing it! It's awful and it's sad. It's emotional, exciting, dramatic, tense. Death is something that just can't happen. The nurses are so competent, not one wasted moment.*

8:48 P.M.

The lights of the sleepy college town are visible as Moston radios, "Gainesville tower, this is Lifeguard 45 Charlie Poppa. Request final landing instructions."

8:55 P.M.

At MCV, nurses Beeston, Parish, and Witherington finish their preparations for surgery. At the Operating Room Command Post, Jane Evanchyk, in turn, calls intensive care. "We're ready. Send up the patient." Next she informs the blood bank, "We're going to surgery with the liver transplant."

Capt. Moston taxis the Lear up to the blocks at Hangar One. Eltonhead opens the hatch, and Posner, Alspaugh, and Mills run to the waiting ambulance from Shands Hospital. On the way to the ambulance, Diana gets the telephone number at the hangar so she can contact Eltonhead during the operation. With lights blazing and sirens screaming, the ambulance shatters the calm of the quiet winter evening as it rushes the recovery team to the hospital. Moston and Eltonhead wait in the lobby of Hangar One, refuel the plane, and arrange for catering. The pilots know time is critical. Everything must be ready when the team comes screaming back with its precious cargo.

9:00 P.M.

At the hospital in Gainesville, the organ procurement officer repositions his patient and administers chest physiotherapy. The teenager's still breathing. Bill knows the next several hours are critical. He also obtains a complete blood count and finishes an hourly monitoring of intake and output. He'll be taking the brain-dead youngster to the OR in an hour.

In Richmond, Cheryl Wood completes her final pre-op check list. Her last entry on the chart that goes to the OR reads, "patient wearing 2 religious bracelets, one on left and the other on right. Patient wishes these to be left on."

Two young men from the transport department arrive to take the patient to surgery. Accompanied by Cheryl Wood, the team begins the trip to the operating room. Retta, Jay, Joan, and Janet watch with a mixture of resignation, relief, exhaustion. After years of fielding international phone calls and after fifteen intense hours this day, Retta is numb as she watches the proceedings.

9:05 P.M.

Posner, Alspaugh, and Mills reach Shands Hospital and learn that although the kidney team is local, the heart team is coming in from

Birmingham. They—the liver team—must wait an hour before starting recovery. Mills worries, because some recovery teams are not really prompt at all, and time is crucial. She and Posner stew. Diana calls Eltonhead at Hangar One and Christy at MCV with a revised timetable: enter the OR at 10 p.m. and ETA at the plane 12:30 to 1 a.m. Meanwhile, Posner is studying the charts.

9:10 P.M.

In the MRICU, the doors of Room 513 swing open and the transport team and the nurses begin the trip upstairs. As the group enters the surgery area, Christy Heindl, at the phone relying messages from the recovery team, gets her first look at the face belonging to the name she has seen on the computer monitor screen in the procurement office for six long months. It's not a pleasant sight. *He looks horrible, thin, sort of like he could glow in the dark. What an odd color, a kind of grey-orange. They'd better hurry up and get that liver. It's going take a lot of fancy footwork to get the job done tonight.* She refocuses her attention on the role she must play.

9:15 P.M.

Beeston's two-hour preparation for the surgery is over, and he steps out of the operating room to get his first look at his patient. Although he has already put in a full day, the nurse anesthetist is excited. "When there's a liver going down, it's the only game in town." Beeston moves forward and injects the first pre-anesthesia.

In Gainesville, Posner frets and waits. Normally the operation in Richmond can't begin until he returns with the liver, but tonight will be special because of the critical nature of the patient and because of the portacaval shunt complications. Mendez will need more time than usual. The delay may mean that Mendez will have to open his patient before Posner removes the donor liver. The young surgeon knows that would be a big gamble. He's glad he doesn't have to make that decision.

Next he worries about the recovery itself. He knows several different medical teams will be working in the operating room at the same time. His thoughts wander. *Sometimes cooperating is not so easy. I hope we don't have one of those crazy heart teams who want to pour ice water on the heart at the moment of harvest. Water's all over everybody and there's two inches of water on the floor. I have to interact*

with different teams from different programs, and sometimes they are
touchy and have their own ideas of how to do it. Sometimes it's not so
easy. Who's going to be here tonight? Is he going to give me a hard
time? Will the kidney guy get insulted if I sort of do his thing if I don't
have time to wait for him? Posner and Mendez confer on the phone and
plot further strategy. Mendez knows that his patient is ready to enter the
OR. Mendez has several hours before he must begin the surgery.
Perhaps by that time Posner will know more.

9:26 P.M.

In Richmond, it's time for the final few steps to the OR. The
transport team completes its job by wheeling its patient twenty yards
straight ahead, where a left turn moves the group into the west wing
toward Operating Room 15. Across the way are units 14 and 16, where
heart transplants are done. None is scheduled tonight. The donor heart
and kidneys are going elsewhere.

The double doors to #15 open. The room itself is rather ordinary,
especially in light of the high-tech surgery that takes place here. As the
members of the team enter the room, which is about twenty-four feet
square, they see the clock on the far wall and, on the left, x-rays and
films of the myriad tests done in the pre-transplant evaluation. The
information is displayed so the surgeons can see everything from their
position on the right of the table. As the surgeon faces the patient, he can
see all the displays by looking straight ahead. By turning his head left,
he can see a TV monitor mounted over the door, which enables him to
view, in a quick glance, various heart functions, wave forms for the
electrocardiogram, all pressure tracings, arterial blood pressure, and
pulmonary artery blood pressure. The wall behind the surgeons has a
series of cabinets and cupboards, not unlike what one might see in a
kitchen. The patient is in the room aligned in a north-south direction,
with the surgeon on the patient's right and the anesthesia team at the
head of the table, separated from the action by a chest-level drape.

The room is jammed with high-tech machinery: the anesthesia
machine, the Rapid Infusion system (for blood transfusions), a cell-
washing device, and a machine to monitor saturation of the venous
blood, plus a special cart of instruments designed specifically for the
transplant and a blue cart for anesthesiology, with drugs, intertracheal
tubes, needles, extensions, labels, syringes. In addition, four pumps are

clamped on a double IV pole that altogether holds four IVs. Two large tables at the foot of the patient are laden with the instruments for the operation.

The journey from the MRICU over, the transport team turns its patient over to the OR staff. Gathered in the room at the time are the anesthesiology team, two doctors, attending Dr. Shribman, resident Dr. Albert; nurse anesthetist, John Beeston; scrub nurse, Debbie Grant; circulating nurse, Barbara Parish; and two perfusionists for blood transfusions, Sandy Witherington and Ty Aaron.

9:30 P.M.

Barbara Parish receives the patient, and Debbie secures him to the operating table with a seat belt-like device across the thighs and arms. Barbara turns on the warming blanket. Draping and preparation for surgery begin.

In the MCV parking lot, Joan, Jay, Retta, and Janet say an emotional farewell and prepare to return home.

9:32 P.M.

Beeston places a blood pressure cup on the left arm, attaches three wires for the electrocardiogram, and another device that measures how well the blood is being oxygenated.

9:40 P.M.

The anesthesiology team is moving rapidly to put its charge to sleep. Beeston slips a mask over the patient's face, turns the head up ten degrees, and administers a drug through the IV that brings unconsciousness quickly, but does nothing to suppress the heart. Next comes the "killer" drug, which creates a state of total paralysis. Almost immediately there is absolutely no muscle function left anywhere in the body. This is done in extreme surgery to still all movement while the surgeons are doing their delicate cutting and suturing.

A machine now takes over the human function of breathing. The machine assumes a kind of life of its own; without it, the human being lying motionless on the table is dead. The blue anesthesiology machine with all its gauges and dials is breathing for a human being. It maintains life mechanically, enabling the doctors to do artificially what the body does every mini-second naturally, without ever thinking. All of this expensive and valuable machinery is in a mini microchip of the brain. Beeston puts tape over the eyes of the body, which is unable to sustain its own life. A human being becomes a machine. The surgical gown comes off.

9:45 P.M.

A floor below, Cheryl Wood is supervising efforts to prepare the room in the MRICU for the patient's return. Housekeeping is already in the room scrubbing, cleaning, and disinfecting walls, floors, and ceiling. This precaution is necessary only in liver transplant patients. Cheryl affixes the name plate to the bed, orders fifty preprinted labels, and an isolation cart, and places an isolation sign on the door.

In OR #15, the anesthesiology team completes placing the tubes in the trachea and makes final adjustments to the machine. Witherington and Aaron prepare the perfusion machine, which allows the blood to be moved to the patient much more rapidly than with the normal slow drip from traditional 300 cc blood bags. Often in transplant surgery, a patient can lose a liter of blood in a fraction of a second. They load the four liters that are always kept ready.

9:55 P.M.

Anesthesiology is inserting tubes. Shribman locates the internal jugular vein and inserts two lines. One will go through the right chamber of the heart (the right ventricle) and to the lung. Other lines have ports that go to the perfusion team for transfusion. The perfusionists are now carefully checking the blood, making sure each unit has "John Robbins, AB positive 5666857H7043" written on it.

Beeston moves to work on the wrist while Shribman is working on the neck. Beeston is starting a line in both arms. Suddenly he gets his first sight of the strings. *God I've heard about these things before*, he thinks. He tells his colleagues, "Ann Reid said, 'When John Robbins comes, don't do anything to those strings.' 'What happens if they are in the way?' I asked. 'I don't know,' she said, 'but don't cut them off.'" Beeston is relieved to find that the strings are tied loosely around the wrists. He carefully pushes them about three inches up each arm, tapes them down, and continues inserting lines in the wrist. When he completes his work, he realizes that the team has now inserted five lines in the patient. They are behind schedule.

10:00 P.M.

In the darkness of the ride back up Interstate 95, Retta and Janet are passing the signs for the closed Kings Dominion amusement park. "Whew" is the feeling in the car. Janet remarks, "Now he's in the hands of the people who know what they are doing, and everything will go according to plan." A well-executed plan lies at the center of Janet's Capricorn life.

"I thought the critical thing was getting John out of Mary Washington fast. He's safe at MCV." Retta agrees with Janet. The efficiency and calmness of Ann Reid and her team had reassured Retta.

Jay, driving another car, is not so sure. He tells Joan, "I haven't seen the liver yet. It's not here, and they say they're going to transplant him. It's such a risk. His chances are so slim. I just don't know."

In Gainesville, the OR supervisor calls the organ procurement officer to bring the patient to surgery. He's kept the teenager breathing on the machine with blood circulating for four critical hours. Two more hours should be enough.

Meanwhile, Marc Posner is assessing the situation to himself. *The donor can arrest* [stop breathing] *the minute I walk in the operating room, or I can be halfway through the procurement and not anywhere near a good position to complete the harvest and the donor craps out. I've lost the liver and Mendez will have Robbins open and we have no more options. I want to be quick, hurry up and get the liver out of here before anything happens.*

10:10 P.M.

The MCV team of Posner, Alspaugh, and Mills enter the OR in Gainesville. They find the teenage donor, the organ procurement official, two nurses from Shands, a kidney preservationist technician, the heart and kidney teams, and the anesthesiologist, who maintains oxygenation and monitors blood pressure. Thirteen people—nurses, doctors, and technicians—are working in the room.

10:15 P.M.

Posner lifts his scalpel and makes the first incision. The harvest is underway. Diana calls Christy at MCV.

10:30 P.M.

Janice Rossi leaves her house in Richmond's Southside and prepares for her trip to MCV to relieve Barbara Parish in the OR. As she drives down Semmes Avenue heading for the Manchester Bridge, she thinks, *This is a liver. I'm in for a long time and I'm going to take a lot of heat. I don't feel like putting up with that tonight.*

10:45 P.M.

Dr. Shribman from anesthesiology looks up at the clock. His team has completed its task before 11 p.m. Good time, considering the difficulty that the frequently invaded veins of the patient presented. All lines are now in place, and surgery can begin. The word is passed to Mendez. At this moment, he receives a call from his young protégé in Gainesville and knows that his colleague has opened the donor, but has not yet dissected the liver. So far the donor appears stable. It will be an hour and a half at a minimum before the liver is out, and at least another three and a half before it can reach Richmond.

The pressure turns up to an even higher level. The drama reaches a new plateau. The Spaniard hesitates. He wonders. He examines alternatives. Should he go ahead now? Should he wait? Timing is always a major decision in transplant, from the very moment a patient is evaluated. At what point in the process should the doctors attempt very risky surgery that may well deprive someone of months of life if it is not successful? If, on the other hand, he waits too long, the patient may die waiting for the transplant. The coma obviated that choice, but presented another difficult one of timing. When should he begin? The cocky Mendez believes that now—at 10:45 p.m., Thursday the twelfth of February, 1987—his patient is already past the point of no return. He considers the moment of incision for someone in coma tantamount to crossing the Rubicon in liver transplant surgery. He can't turn back now. *Alea jacta est.* The die is cast, the Rubicon crossed.

Mendez needs more time than usual because of the complications of the shunt. He'll wait a little longer. But how much longer? So far the timing has been precise, almost miraculous. The hour delay he built into his first calculations has, however, already been used up by the wait getting into the operating room in Gainesville. There are bound to be some more surprises once he opens up the patient. He has to have a margin.

He decides to go into the OR in half an hour, well before Posner finishes the harvest. He'll open up less than an hour before Thursday the twelfth turns into Friday the thirteenth. The gamble must be taken. The life of his patient depends on the accuracy of his judgment. It's an awesome responsibility. It's a life-or-death gamble. A life lies in the skilled hands and the sound judgment of the forty-two-year-old whiz of transplant surgery.

11:00 P.M.

Nurse Janice Rossi slips into the OR to relieve Barbara Parish. She finds the room fairly quiet. No one has yet turned on the music. Parish has, however, stocked the room with the music the surgeons like. Mendez can operate in silence, while Posner likes classical music. Beethoven is ready for his arrival from Gainesville. Rossi thinks that Mendez's screaming during the first part of the operation will provide enough music and decides not to turn on more noise. Mendez will be under unusual pressure until the portacaval shunt is dissected. That will be music enough.

Nurse Willie Artist arrives with Rossi to replace Debbie Grant. The surgical intern Loundrey enters and begins final preparations for Mendez's arrival. He takes the drape back and begins painting the surgical area with an antiseptic.

11:13 P.M.

Perfusionist Ty Aaron adds the first 200 cc of blood to the machine because blood loss, accompanied by the dilating of the vessels due to anesthesia, drops the level of blood and makes the heart beat faster. To lower the rapidly beating heart, blood is transfused. Rapid loss of blood and the resulting strain on the heart is one of the prime dangers in liver transplant surgery.

A greater than normal amount of blood-loss for a liver transplant will be the case tonight because of previous surgery, the portacaval shunt, performed sixteen months ago in Bangkok. Shribman's team must monitor the pressure carefully throughout the hours of the operation.

11:15 P.M.

The doors to the operating room open. A new atmosphere pervades the room. Mendez strides in confidently. He is assertive in the operating room and has thought through everything very carefully. Tonight he knows what he wants to do and what he must do to accomplish his goal. He has made his plans and considered his fallback positions. He is in charge, and everyone knows it from the moment he enters the room. He surveys the scene, advances to the table like a potentate. He is the unquestioned master. "Good evening. How are you? This is going to be tough, ladies and gentlemen. Because of the patient's previous surgery, he has lots of scar tissue. In addition, he had almost no clotting factors and no platelets when he arrived at the OR. We have to do a lot of cutting before we can get to the dissection. You put all of those factors together, and you know we are going to have a long operation with a lot of bleeding."

11:25 P.M.
Posner splits the sternum, gets his first look at the donor liver, and calls MCV. Next, he begins the dissection of the structures in the free edge of the lesser omentum to prepare the way for the dissection and removal of the liver. He places silk slings around the dissected structures—the coeliac, splenic, common hepatic and gastroduodenal arteries, the portal vein, and the common bile duct.

11:30 P.M.
Beeston reads off blood pressure 120/65, heart rate 75. Everything stable.

11:32 P.M.
"Knife!" Thoughts rush through the surgeon's mind. *I don't know if this patient is going to survive. I feel it to a higher degree tonight because the coma has complicated what I know surgically is going to be a hell of a challenge.* Putting his thoughts behind him, Mendez begins the incision, which goes along the middle of the chest from the top of the breastbone to an inch or so above the navel and off in a semicircle on both sides towards the hips. The surgeon is outward bound.

The operation begins. Now he must loosen the organs, dissect the liver and portacaval shunt, and hope he can get it all done with enough time left to sew in the donor liver. He also has to hope Posner does not run into serious problems and that the weather holds so the plane can return with the liver.

The surgeon steels his will and reassures himself. *I have doubts, but I've made the decision not to wait and to go in now, because that's the best thing to do for the patient. I'm very involved, but if I don't get so involved every time I go into the operating room, I'm not doing the best for my patient.* Mendez is tense, but he knows that seconds from now the tension will dissipate, and he will be totally involved in saving a life and breaking medical barriers.

Heart rate jumps up and blood pressure drops twenty points. Beeston notes low arterial pressure and calls for increased transfusion. As blood pressure drops and the machine gets behind in volume, heart rate goes up, because it is trying to get whatever blood is left around faster. Pulmonary diastolic pressure now governs transfusion rate.

The anesthesia team is making decisions about how much blood to put in and when. Beeston turns to the perfusionists. "Open the lines and give us 200 cc of blood." The perfusionist works with the anesthesiologist in response to the numbers on the anesthesia machine. Bleeding is heavy; clotting is poor because the liver is in such bad shape.

The blood's clotting factors are produced in the liver, and when the organ is functioning at minimum capacity, bleeding is, and remains, a constant threat in the transplant. Thus, a damaged liver makes any operation more difficult, especially a liver transplant, because it's a bloody procedure. One-quarter of the body's blood supply goes to the liver with each heartbeat. The poor clotting is one of the factors that makes a liver transplant more difficult and more tricky than heart and kidney transplants. In addition, because the liver performs so many separate and vital functions in the body, nothing can take its place. This puts the liver transplant surgeon under an unusual time stress. He must complete his work in a very narrow time-frame since—unlike for the heart and kidneys—no machine can take over for the liver. All these factors combine to make a very tense time. The slightest hesitation in getting an instrument can set off a stream of curses in the Mendez operating room.

11:48 P.M.

The incision is complete and the real meat of the surgery is now beginning. Mendez turns his attention to dissecting the portacaval shunt that Dr. Chanvit constructed sixteen months ago in Bangkok. Tension mounts as Mendez forges ahead into new territory.

After the incision, Mendez begins to break down and isolate the blood vessels going to the liver. In a normal person, one who does not have cirrhosis, this is a fairly easy task. Previous surgery makes it more difficult because of scar tissue. In addition, often other organs are stuck and difficult to move.

11:50 P.M.

Yelling begins. Nurse Rossi knows "there's always a lot of yelling in a transplant. Suctions aren't working fast enough, and if it takes you two seconds to go to the corner to get something, the surgeons don't understand why you can't have everything on the table at the same time. Mendez yells when things are not going right." Rossi has explained this to nursing students many times. "What scares nurses inexperienced in liver transplants is that they don't know the seriousness of the operation. They don't know the tension is going to be high and they run the risk of getting yelled at—not because they've done anything wrong, but just because it's a pressure-filled, life-and-death situation. You can't always control what goes on: blood pressure can fall, the patient can bleed, the patient can go into arrest, and things are happening so quickly that you don't always have time to recognize what is going on. Transplants are long. You are on your feet a long time. You have to be fast and attentive. You really have to think on your feet, and if you just happen to be a little slow, you run the risk of getting yourself yelled at."

The perfusionists add 500 cc of blood to compensate for blood lost during incision. Mendez is working furiously and quickly as he confronts complications that have foiled a host of the world's best liver transplant surgeons. The tension gripping the operating room now comes from Mendez—"my sense of responsibility, my sense of commitment to my patient. I go crazy when things don't go well. I really can't take it."

He knows the major problems of liver transplant surgery are ahead of him—unforeseen complications in taking out the liver, problems with the donor. And hemorrhage remains one of the greatest dangers in transplant surgery. Despite all efforts and even with the most careful dissection and suturing of all bleeding vessels, there may be spontaneous hemorrhage when the abdomen is opened. There is a constant problem with air embolus, because if the central venous pressure falls unexpectedly and there is a defect in the vena cava, air may be sucked into the right side of the heart, killing the patient. Always there is the fear of over-transfusion, by following a too-vigorous attempt to replace real or estimated blood loss. Finally, as more cyclosporine is added during the operation to guard against rejection, the patient runs the risk of kidney failure. Mendez understands all of this, worries, but settles into the operation and forges ahead.

4

...a time to break down,
a time to build up...

It's midnight and a hectic Thursday, February twelfth, turns into Friday the thirteenth. The battle against all odds for a new life has been unfolding for eighteen hours in many locations scattered throughout the southeastern United States.

In Gainesville and Richmond, doctors Posner and Mendez are in crucial phases of surgery. Posner operates on a brain-dead teenager whose vital organs have been donated to preserve life, and Mendez works on a critically ill patient in a desperate effort to defy death and create a new life. A plane is fueled and ready. One surgeon is near the crucial moment of organ retrieval; the other is at the most tense moment of the opening phase of his surgery. The night is quiet and still. The principal elements of the drama are playing out almost a thousand miles apart.

12:15 A.M.

Mendez, in the midst of dissecting the portacaval shunt, is "scared beyond belief that all of sudden, I am going to find that nothing can be done to save my patient." His major fears are either that the scar tissue will be so extensive he won't be able to separate other organs to remove the diseased liver or that the portal vein—one of the major suppliers of blood to the liver—will be so short that he won't be able to repair it.

133

How good was Dr. Chanvit's surgery in Bangkok? The volatile Spaniard has been working furiously and quickly for half an hour. "I've told you four times already to give me this . . . what am I talking to? The wall?" As he continues delicate moves in the early, tense phase of the operations, he screams at the defenseless scrub nurse, "What is this?!! A smorgasbord?!! A serve-yourself operating room? Please give me help!" And then another "*Help me!*" several decibels louder, punctuated with a string of expletives. The surgeon looks over the curtain to anesthetist John Beeston and says, "How does that sound?"

"Fine," Beeston smiles back. He is familiar with Mendez's operating-room style.

12:20 A.M.

Another string of expletives followed by, "Watch me! The operation is *here*, not over there on the *goddamn wall.*" Mendez's explosions are normal for a tense operating room. He rationalizes, "All surgeons yell. I have never seen one who doesn't, unless he does bunions or ingrown toenails for a living. My yelling is my Spanish temperament, and it is my relief valve."

Suddenly the surgeon turns excitedly to the intern, Loundrey, and exclaims with relief and pride, "Gee, it doesn't look that tough. . . . Gee, that's a well-made portacaval shunt. . . . The Thai doctor did a good job. . . . I think we have it. I think we have it." Mendez is exuberant. Perhaps the shunt is not going to be the great stumbling block after all. Thirty or forty minutes into the operation, the colorful surgeon has reached his operating "high." He thinks, *Wow, he's going to be done. God bless, there's no question about it. We're going to do it.* Although he is excited, he begins to slow down. Once the great fear is over, he begins to pace himself, because he knows he's got more time. He can't sustain his opening pace. He is like a basketball coach who begins a game in a full-court press and fast break—a supercharged, hectic, emotional game plan. When he suddenly realizes his team is in control, and the game can be won, he orders his charges to slow down. He knows they have to keep up the pressure, but he feels, *Gosh, these guys aren't so tough; we can beat them. All we've go to do is play our game now, and not get exhausted.* Mendez knows this feeling because he has reached this point in the transplant game.

While Mendez is exulting in Richmond, Posner's harvest on the teenager in Gainesville is reaching its critical stage. The scene in the Gainesville OR is tense. Three surgeons, three prima donnas, three ballerinas of medicine are prancing around the table, each one absolutely convinced he and his methods are the best. Curses are usually swallowed here. The talk is often strained and overly polite. Posner, ordinarily almost as volatile in the operating room as Mendez, remains quiet. He works quickly:

The branches of the left gastric artery are tied and divided.

The lesser omentum is dissected further.

The gall bladder is mobilized from its bed.

The right kidney is mobilized and lifted forward.

Slings are placed around the renal vein and the vena cava.

12:25 A.M.

The heart surgeons move forward to harvest the heart. *Are these jokers going to pour water over everyone?* Posner wonders to himself. No water! The heart harvested, life-support turned off, the teenager stops breathing. Posner rushes in to finish harvesting the liver. He prepares to complete all the dissections so the liver can be lifted from the body.

12:30 A.M.

While Mendez has slowed down, Posner is stepping up his pace to get the liver free and back to Richmond. First he has to clean and cool the organ by stopping the blood flow and adding preservatives that will allow the body's largest internal organ to remain functional so it can be preserved and brought back to Richmond. He connects tubes to various parts of the liver and threads another tube into the all-important portal vein. Finally in this stage, he separates the liver from its major blood supply, meaning that arterial blood now circulates through the tubes from the aorta, not through the liver itself. Blood circulation almost ceases. The diaphragm is cut in front of the vena cava, and the inferior vena cava above the liver is divided. The dissection complete, Posner removes the liver and places it in a bowl of ice-cold saline solution. It's 12:30 a.m. Six hours are available to fly this vital organ back to Richmond and sew it into another body. The clock now joins bleeding and infection as enemies to be overcome.

Advised of Posner's progress, Mendez is, at this same moment, completing his dissection so he can cut the diseased liver out of his patient within moments after Posner returns to the MCV operating room with the teenager's donated liver.

Posner carries the new liver, with the tubes still attached, to the back table and begins perfusing solutions through the organ, which will cool it down and preserve it for about six hours. He and Diana Mills, from the MCV procurement office, are working rapidly, because every second is of utmost importance. The quicker the liver can be sewed into its new body, the greater are the chances that it will function properly—and Robbins' prospects for survival will increase dramatically. But as time outside the body approaches six hours, the risk that the new liver will fail becomes greater. Every minute can become a lifetime. All those involved in the transplant effort at this moment—doctors, nurses, pilots, drivers, everyone—understand this and turn up their effort and concentration a notch. As in a crucial basketball game, it's crunch time. It's the moment when a mental error can cost you the game. Except in the game of transplant, a mental error costs a life.

Posner and Mills work rapidly to prepare the organ for its trip. Posner inserts the cooled and perfused liver into a bowl of fresh saline solution that, in turn, is doubled-bagged in sterile polythene containers of iced saline solution. Finally, this bag, which contains a last hope for a man's life, is placed on ice in a Styrofoam container. It rides to its rendezvous with destiny in an Igloo cooler, much like those lugged to football games, races, the beach, and picnics.

12:45 A.M.

Diana Mills calls First Officer Eltonhead at the plane. "We're on our way." She makes an identical call to her colleague from the MCV procurement office, who answers the telephone outside the OR in Richmond. Posner, Mills, and Alspaugh shed their OR scrubs and head for the ambulance, which now screams through town on its way to the airport.

12:55 A.M.

Posner, Alspaugh, and Mills take their seats on the Lear, and Moston calls the tower for taxi instructions. He hears, "Roger, Lifeguard 45 Charlie Poppa. Taxi to runway one five."

Mendez now faces the vena cava, the major vein that carries blood back from the legs and the lower part of the body to the heart. The vena cava's position in the body presents the major obstacle to removing the liver while, at the same time, preserving the patient's cardiac function. As he moves to clear the obstacle that the vena cava presents, the surgeon gets his first view of the diseased liver, now a shrunken cirrhotic organ after years of ravaging by hepatitis B virus. He moves his quick hands to the omentum, a strong, colorless, smooth membrane that goes from the stomach to other organs. Its structures must be carefully separated from each other and controlled by slings. He slips a green silk loop around the bile duct, a blue one around the portal vein, and a red one around the common hepatic artery.

1:00 A.M.

"Gainesville Tower, this is Lifeguard 45 Charlie Poppa, ready for takeoff, runway two zero."

"Roger, cleared for takeoff."

1:03 A.M.

"Departure, this is Lifeguard 45 Charlie Poppa at a thousand."

"Roger, cleared to climb to niner thousand, turn right heading two four zero." The new liver is airborne and on its way back up the Eastern seaboard to Richmond. Weather is clear, and Eltonhead anticipates no problems ahead.

In the operating room, Mendez is well into his last steps of taking out the liver. He clamps and divides the ligamentum teres, a V-shaped fibrous band attached to various ligaments that have to be moved to get the liver out. He clamps and divides all of the ligaments and other attachments that anchor the liver in the body. Next, he elevates the liver and bends down so he can make the final sutures and divide the adrenal vein. *He's finished.*

Now he makes an incision and inserts tubes in the right groin and the inner upper right arm. This will enable blood to be routed around the area of the liver during the time the organ is out of the body, while the new liver is being sewn in.

Capt. Moston radios the Atlanta Center that he has reached his cruising altitude of 38,000 feet. He tells Diana that the estimated time of arrival in Richmond is 2:45 a.m. Diana, in turn, calls Christy,who alerts the surgical team at MCV.

1:30 A.M.

Mendez is now finishing the opening stage of the surgery. He arranges tubes and places packs to absorb bleeding. Beeston writes on the chart, "packed off awaiting donor organ." Mendez leaves the operating room. The unknown phase of the operation is behind. From now on the transplant is "routine." It has taken two hours to reach this stage, an hour longer than normal. He has, however, reached this goal with about an hour and a half to spare. So far his timing is perfect. Barring a complication with the plane, he is going to have enough time to sew in the new liver and still meet the 6:30 a.m. deadline. The part of the operation he had hyped himself for—dissecting the portacaval shunt—is now over, but the "meat" of the operation—putting in the liver—remains. He leaves his patient "comfortably bleeding" in the OR and retreats to the lounge for a little time off his feet. Anesthesiology is now in charge of the OR.

Mendez, relaxing over a cup of coffee, explains, "John will not survive if something happens to that donor liver. We are talking about liver reserve. Some patients can be opened up, have everything dissected and prepared to take the liver, and their reserve still makes them able to tolerate that insult even if the liver doesn't arrive. Robbins can't do that. No question about it, because his reserve is zero. His liver was working at capacity to keep him alive, and whatever he summoned to stay alive before the operation, he doesn't have any more."

A floor below, critical care nurse Cheryl Wood finishes preparing and stocking the room in the MRICU, awaiting the end of surgery. She has completed a checklist of two and a half pages, numbering forty-eight items and over a hundred separate duties. Her long day over, Cheryl heads for home. The room looks like a scene from Star Trek.

2:40 A.M.

Aboard Lifeguard 45 Charlie Poppa, everything looks right on schedule. Capt. Moston turns to the radio, contacts Richmond approach, identifies himself, and requests final landing instructions.

2:44 A.M.

Moston guides the Lear 35 into its blocks at Hawthorne Aviation at Richmond's Byrd Airport. First Officer Eltonhead opens the hatch, and Posner, lugging the Igloo cooler with its precious cargo, trailed by Mills and Alspaugh, runs for the transplant car, which is warmed and ready. They turn on the flashing lights so as not to waste a second getting into the city. Every moment assumes a critical life of its own.

2:55 A.M.

The Richmond skyline pops out of the darkness as the transplant car rushes into the city. The lights of the old MCV tower appear on the left. The car hurtles across Shokoe Bottoms, bordering the James River, exits left to Canal Street, goes one more block. Now the Richmond Coliseum is on the right. Another right turn brings the group past the White House of the Confederacy. Then a left and the car reaches the MCV emergency entrance. Posner runs in, gripping the cooler. The liver has reached MCV.

3:00 A.M.

Posner rushes into the OR and the room is immediately filled up with questions:

"How did it go?"

"Good flight?"

"Is it a big liver?"

"How's it look?"

Weariness slips away. Excitement and anticipation dominate for the moment. The seriousness of the situation gives way to some lighthearted comments. There is, however, little time for banter. Very serious work lies ahead. The banter does not supplant the work; it merely goes along with it.

3:05 A.M.

Mendez moves forward confidently. The room stills for a moment, and only the whir of the hundreds of thousands of dollars worth of high-tech equipment can be heard. Deftly, the Spanish surgeon places a clamp on the portal vein. Next he clamps the hepatic artery and the intrahepatic vena cava. The room stills even more as the tension rises. The perfusionists and the anesthesiologists ready themselves. Soon the machine that has been breathing for the patient is joined by another that circulates blood outside the body so the old, diseased liver can come out and the lifegiving new one can be sewn into place.

Mendez turns to Nurse Artist and yells, "Clamp." It is placed firmly in his hand, and he uses it on the suprahepatic inferior vena cava. It takes a bite out of the diaphragm and keeps the vena cava from slipping during the removal of the old and the sewing in of the new liver. The surgeon clamps the vena cava, the portal vein, and the hepatic artery, and cuts the common bile duct.

The stage is now set for veno-veno bypass—forcing the blood to circulate outside the body while the liver is removed and its replacement is sewn in. During the initial stage of this move, the body will lose approximately forty percent of its blood volume. When the body is on full veno-veno bypass, blood is taken from the inferior vena cava at the femoral vein in the right thigh, run through the pump, and returned to the superior vena cava through the incision made earlier in the brachial vein of the right forearm.

The room hushes. The perfusionists turn their full attention to the dials of their machine. As blood flows, it must maintain a certain rate so it doesn't form clots. When blood circulates outside the body, the revolutions per minute of the perfusion machine must be greater than a liter per minute to keep cardiac output and blood pressure from dropping and the blood from forming clots. When Mendez hears one thousand or more, he knows the flow rate is safe and he can make his final cut. Mendez turns to Beeston. "What's the flow rate?"

"Two thousand."

3:06 A.M.

These words initiate veno-veno by pass, the crucial phase of the operation. The clamps are closed, and the blood bypasses the vena cava. Mendez readies himself to cut out the diseased liver. Transplant surgery is now unfolding with a rhythm all its own. It is, in the words of Posner, "The quintessential technical exercise. You have to have technical expertise, good judgment, patience. The surgeon must plan well and anticipate all problems. The technical part of it is very demanding. Liver transplant is the biggest operation you can possibly do to anybody, because it takes longer, requires more stamina, and involves time constraints. I can do other procedures, and I'm not racing the clock. But you take the liver out of the ice, put it in the patient, start to sew it in, and you don't have time to re-do it. It all has to be done in a short period of time or it isn't going to work."

3:07 A.M.

Two surgeons—Posner and Mendez—move at full speed as the operation steps up another notch in intensity. Words are short and curt.

"This stitch here."

"That stitch there."

"The bitch won't stop bleeding."

Both surgeons are working furiously. Although "they fit equally in supportive roles . . . a collegial thing" (Beeston's words), there's only one quarterback. That's Mendez.

Two surgeons, at work simultaneously, make the liver transplant particularly difficult for everyone else. Both surgeons bark an incessant flow of commands to the beleaguered nurses, whose woes as a result are doubled. Two bosses, both demanding, expecting demands to be met quickly. Thus for a nurse, the liver transplant is not only long, but also it's double trouble, double tension, double yelling.

3:08 A.M.

Mendez cuts the hepatic artery and the vena cava above and below the liver. The all-out sprint against the clock, testing the skills of the surgeon to defy nature, begins in earnest. No machine stands ready to perform the liver's myriad tasks. There is no fallback position. It is now all or nothing at all. A new life . . . or death.

3:18 A.M.

A 1000 cc (about twenty percent of the body's capacity) more of blood are added in less than ten minutes. The operation is really reaching its bloody phase.

3:20 A.M.

Gently, Mendez removes the liver. The diseased organ, whose failure has brought the patient to near-death, lies in a basin outside his body, awaiting its final journey to pathology. Mendez and Posner have three hours to sew in the teenager's healthy liver, which is lying in an iced saline solution several yards behind the operating table.

3:30 A.M.

The perfusionists add another 700 cc of blood. At this moment, the liver has been out of its first body for three hours. Mendez has reached the halfway point on schedule. The major obstacles of repairing the portal vein (damaged by the portacaval shunt) and sewing in the new liver remain. Recognizing his enormous challenge, Mendez moves quickly to begin the final stage of getting the portal vein in the proper position, so he can begin the process of sewing in the new liver before too much more time elapses. If he can get this next step done, sew in the liver, and come in under the 6:30 a.m. deadline, his patient might just make it.

Mendez is not happy with what he finds. The portal vein is normally straight, but the shunt puts a bend in it. Getting the vein straight is important, because the portal vein is the major supplier of the blood to the liver. The liver cannot function properly without a good supply of blood.

The surgeon's frustration reaches a high level as he can't get the vein to stay straight. He remarks to no one in particular, in his best Latin accent, "How! The bitch won't stay straight." It takes him several more attempts and fallback moves to get the vein in the right position so he can begin sewing in the new liver.

He continues making moves, cursing and sewing. The bleeding is heavy and the perfusion team is constantly readying more blood. Mendez summons all the skill he gained in over thirty previous liver transplants, countless vascular surgeries, and kidney transplants to compel the operation to go his way, to make him the master, the controller, not a reactor. The transplant has reached the stage that calls upon Mendez's vaunted ability for split-second decisions and quick, sure reactions. He knows the surgeon cannot panic. If it won't work one way, try another. Quickly but methodically, Mendez fashions a way to keep the vein in shape and make it stay straight.

4:00 A.M.

The body has been without its largest internal organ for forty minutes. It probably cannot go more than a total of three hours without a liver. The portacaval shunt complications have eaten up thirty to forty-five minutes, and the operation is running that far behind. Nevertheless, Mendez is not overly concerned at this juncture. But the operating room seems to pause. The banter stops. There is one collective holding of breath as Mendez and Posner remove the donor liver from the ice and begin the process of sewing it in the body. The operation reaches its crucial and most intense moment. The surgeons hope there will be no more complications. Mendez simply doesn't have time for new problems.

The two surgeons work together to place cuffs on the surface of the new liver and around the superhepatic inferior vena cava. The suturing reaches a furious pace as the two surgeons begin the process of joining vessels to sew in the new organ. Mendez skillfully passes a mesiline suture through the extremities of the donor and recipient vena cava. One man's liver is quickly becoming part of another's body. The stitching must be done rapidly, but extraordinarily carefully because of the layers of suturing involved.

4:05 A.M.

The surgeons are totally absorbed in the task of joining the vessels from the new liver to the vessels in its new body. Everyone in the OR recognizes this as a delicate phase of the surgery. The hepatic artery could easily be damaged, resulting in severe clotting and cardiac failure. Mendez completes the suprahepatic inferior vena cava suture and places a small swab between the liver and the clamp so it does not damage the liver during the rest of the operation. Next, he joins the portal veins to make an opening through which the new liver can be perfused, or supplied with blood and warmed.

4:30 A.M.

Everything is going well, and the team can transfuse plasma into the new liver to clean it of the chemicals added to preserve the organ for its trip to Richmond. Over the next eighteen minutes, 1800 cc of blood are added as the surgeons complete the joining of more vessels.

4:54 A.M.

The liver is in! Five major vessels supply the liver with blood and four of the five have now been joined. Mendez takes off the clamps and blood flows through the repaired vessels into the new liver. Blood is once again circulating through the body, as veno-veno bypass ends. Lifegiving blood surges through the new liver and begins the slow process of washing out the fouling preservatives. From a surgical perspective, Mendez is out of the woods. He calls on one of his numerous food analogies to explain the situation. "I have done what is needed. The rest is parsley, potatoes, gravy, but you have the meat."

Mendez is pleased. He starts to sing. The nurses recognize this as an excellent sign. They report that he is "now bouncing off the wall." He knows it's not over yet. The fat lady hasn't sung, though she's getting in tune. A feeling of "Whew, we've done it" pervades the OR. From his first look at the liver fully sewn in the body, Mendez's confidence in the technical success of the surgery soars.

The long road ahead is familiar. He has walked it many times in the past several years. He must wait for the liver to start functioning by making bile, and he understands that he will have another long wait for the bleeding to stop, bleeding due to the many raw surfaces from previous surgery. In addition, many things beyond his technical control could still go wrong.

5:00 A.M.

Beeston looks at the EKG and hollers, "He's fibrillating."

Oh my God, not this, not now after everything with the surgery has gone so well, Mendez thinks. Life is suddenly in jeopardy. The heart, in Mendez's lexicon of food analogies, is "going bananas." He can do nothing about the situation, and if the heart doesn't stop its rapid beating, he knows his patient will die.

For several minutes, Mendez is uncharacteristically quiet. "People die from it all the time in operations. It's tense for me, and I can do nothing about the tension. It's inside, and I don't express it."

It's the anesthesiologists' game to win or lose. Blood pressure, which varied from 125 to 95 during the operation, suddenly drops to 85. The heart rate, which was maintaining in the high 90s, jumps to 130. It's known as an acute ectopic ventriculation. The faster the heart beats, the less time it has to take blood in and expel it. Because the heart has less time to work, the volume of blood supplied to vital organs is reduced. It's a serious, life-threatening situation.

The anesthesiology team reacts rapidly. Shribman looks over at Beeston, and they move quickly to deal with the problem. Beeston gives glucose, insulin, calcium, and one amp of bicarb before the surgeons have time to say anything. It's tense. An eerie silence slips over the room. The machines grind on in their mechanical way. Lines move across the monitors, and a life hangs in the balance.

5:20 A.M.

Blood pressure rises to 100, and the elevated heart rate drops to 82. A collective sign of relief can be heard in operating room 15.

5:30 A.M.

Over the last ten minutes, the perfusionists have added over 2000 cc of blood. To this point in the surgery, blood-loss is above normal even for a liver transplant. The high blood loss is undoubtedly the result of previous surgery, the portacaval shunt, in the same area. The body normally has 5000 cc of blood volume, so every 1000 cc represents twenty percent of the total volume. To this point in the operation, the body has bled out its entire volume of blood. The really bloody part of the ordeal still lies ahead.

Posner and Mendez move to finish the operation. They connect the bile ducts and drains in the new liver. They work on the conduits to the hepatic artery, portal vein, and biliary conduits. Making sure everything is well-stitched, they now look for bleeding points. Finally, they check to see that the liver has a satisfactory appearance and lies in the correct position.

6:00 A.M.

Posner and Mendez finish their vascular work, and the surgery phase of the transplant is over. "The liver looks good," Mendez declares. "Let's warm up the patient, give him fresh frozen, pack it off, and wait. Pour some saline into the belly." Mendez and Posner leave the operating room satisfied. Mendez remarks, "I was damned sure before I began that if I could take the shunt down, I could pull this thing off. Now, with the liver working, it should just be a matter of time. But we have to be persistent and patient. We must not get tired, close, take him to intensive care, and just allow him to bleed in there. I won't do that. We need to be patient."

Despite all of the anticipated complications of the shunt, the surgery itself took only about an hour longer than expected. Mendez and Posner beat the 6:30 a.m. deadline by a full half-hour. They smile as they leave the room. But they don't go far away. Mendez may catch a quick nap.

He wants to look good for his next great performance, the bowing of the virtuoso before the admiring audience. He leaves the OR singing. Posner has his never-changing look—the determined, intense scowl of the angry young man.

5

...a time to mourn,
a time to dance...

The operation, in its ninth hour, has reached a point where the surgical team is waiting for the bleeding to stop and the transplanted liver to give some sign that it is beginning to function in its new body.

6:05 A.M.

With Mendez and Posner having successfully sewn in the donor organ, the long process of warming up the body and cleansing the new liver of the preservatives is now underway.

Transplant places the body in a series of cruel dilemmas. In order for the new liver to be preserved, the organ is stored and transported in an iced saline solution. The icy preservatives, together with anesthesia, have already lowered body temperature to thirty-one or thirty-two degrees centigrade. In this state the body, hibernating like a bear in winter, does not metabolize drugs very well and cannot remove the impurities that have been added to the system. It is locked in a brutal fight with itself. The process of preserving the organ now makes it more difficult for the body to accept its new lifesaving part. Catch 22.

Another problem occurs because, as the body cools, clotting factors in the blood necessary to stem the profuse bleeding go down. The body is cool because it's bleeding, and it's bleeding because it's cool. Catch 44.

The doctors must have a great deal of endurance, and the patient needs a great deal of stamina. The patient, however, has already gone through the most serious shock his system could ever hope to endure. And the doctors have already been in the operating room for over twelve hours. Catch 22 evolves into the plot for a Kafka novel.

From this point forward, throughout the process of the patient's recovery, difficult choices are never far away. At the moment, the most pressing demand is to keep the patient alive, stem the bleeding, close the wound to minimize infection, and get him back to the ICU.

7:00 A.M.

In Fredericksburg, Retta has just awakened and begun to stare at her telephone. *Why doesn't it ring? Ann said she would call, and I haven't heard from her yet.*

8:00 A.M.

Nurse Janice Rossi, after a hectic and loud night, is preparing to leave the OR and turn her duties over to Bennie Casupanan. Mendez has not been too bad tonight, and she has even gotten "Rossi baby," his favorite phrase of endearment, from him a couple of times.

In Fredericksburg, the phone rings. It's Ann Reid. "The surgeons are getting ready to close now. John should be out of the OR soon and Dr. Mendez would like to see you at 11:30." Relieved, Retta relays the encouraging news to Joan and Janet.

9:00 A.M.

The patient is still bleeding heavily in the OR. As a result, the operation is dragging out into its twelfth hour, with the end not yet in sight. In the MCV blood bank, Sally Cook must call Pat Bezak, who is at her office at the Richmond Metropolitan Blood Service. This morning, Cook from MCV and Bezak and Briere from the Blood Service must evaluate the blood supply to make sure the process can continue. A long, bloody operation can sometimes force Briere into a life-or-death judgment.

In his position, Briere has the responsibility for Richmond's blood supply. He never wants to reach a situation in which a transplant has used hundreds of units of blood, so "elective surgery must be canceled or a 19-year-old pregnant girl starts bleeding, and something happens to her because of a diminished blood supply." Briere knows the transplant surgeons "do not want that kind of notoriety. The transplant team does not want to be looked upon as if it is hogging the blood supply." Fortunately this morning, despite the unusually heavy bleeding in last night's transplant, the supply is fine, and Briere gives the word to continue. One more roadblock hurdled.

10:00 A.M.

Because his patient is still bleeding in the OR, Mendez refuses to close.

Diana Mills is awake and calls the OR to check on the status of the transplant.

10:30 A.M.

John Beeston turns to his colleague, Andy Shribman, and says, "The ABGs are going up." This is the best news so far, signaling that the liver is now working, because the patient has just gone from acid to base. The new organ is able to break down and remove citrates in the blood. As the major center for cleansing the body of impurities, it is once again doing one of its hundreds of jobs properly. The light is shining more brightly at the end of the tunnel

Retta gets into her Honda in Fredericksburg and begins the drive to Richmond.

11:30 A.M.

The operation now enters its fourteenth hour. The bleeding continues. Mendez and Posner are back in the OR checking and supervising, looking at stitches and re-doing some sutures. Mendez doesn't want to return his patient to the MRICU if there are still bleeding spots, yet he knows the longer the patient is open and exposed on the table, the risk of infection becomes greater.

Every decision in liver transplant is a trade-off and involves high risks. Should he close and limit the risk of infection? Such a course might, however, increase the danger from internal bleeding and lead to another operation. Close or wait? It's a hard choice for Mendez because he knows that even with the liver working, one of the major dangers ahead is still infection. Nevertheless, he decides to wait a little longer.

Retta arrives at MCV and finds the operation now entering its fifteenth hour. Ann Reid and the other nurses reassure her that nothing is wrong. "The surgeons are just doing little finishing touches." *What could be left following fifteen hours?* she wonders. After yesterday, her faith in the transplant team is great. She settles down to wait.

11:45 A.M.

Joan joins Ret in the small waiting area outside the MRICU. Chris Wood, the primary-care nurse, comes out to reassure them that everything is going well. She reports that Mendez is singing again, so the end must be near. The nurse tells Retta that she has seen the new liver, and it is "beautiful, pink."

NOON

A replacement, Tom Bowman, has now been found for the exhausted nurse anesthetist, John Beeston, who has been at the hospital for the better part of two days.

12:30 P.M.

Mendez and Posner return to the operating room together to see if conditions will permit a closing any time soon. They find that the bleeding is subsiding, the liver is continuing to function well, and the transfusion rate is slowing down. Mendez makes a few more stitches, redoes some sutures, and determines that he might be able to consider closing in two more hours. The operation now enters its sixteenth hour. Each moment longer increases the risk of infection.

1:15 P.M.

A nurse comes out to tell Joan, Retta, and Janet that the operation is going so well that Mendez is "bouncing off the wall. He's on a high because of what he has done. He's still prancing around, but he'll be down to talk to the family in a minute."

2:15 P.M.

Everything looks good to Mendez. He turns to the assistants and says, "Let's get ready to close." He leaves the OR now for his command performance before the family. He showers, changes clothes, and prepares to make his grand entrance in a fresh white jacket—no scrubs for the next show.

2:30 P.M.

The elevator doors on the fourth floor open, and Mendez ambles out casually. Retta remarks to Janet, "He looks crisp, wonderful, as if he had been sleeping for twenty-four hours." He tells the three women, "It's a perfect liver and really fit well. The operation went well. Everything looks fine, and the liver is perfect. Everything seems to be going fine. There were no surprises."

He exudes assurances. Retta feels that he is "very confident" and tells Janet, "Everything has been done right." She finds it hard to believe that something as miraculous as a lifesaving liver transplant, conducted under an emergency situation, can be discussed so routinely by the staff. Mendez tells them what he tells all transplant families: John is "in critical condition, and will remain so for some time to come. The next five days will be crucial, because rejection is still possible at any moment, and there are still many lines that are open roads for infection. But, at this point, the recovery appears routine."

"Is this the first time a transplant has been performed successfully after a portacaval shunt, Dr. Mendez?" Retta asks the surgeon.

"Maybe the first in the world," Mendez replies, "but the procedure is routine among surgical techniques. It is, however, one of the 'of course' procedures."

"What do you mean?" Retta inquires.

"It's like this," the surgeon explains. "This is how I brush my teeth, up and down, sideways. I say that and people generally reply, 'Well, yes, of course, that's normal.' So if you brush your teeth on the top of the Himalayas, you do it the normal way. You don't do it any different. The techniques used are nothing extraordinary.

"But, you see, most people don't generally brush their teeth on the top of the Himalayas." Mendez smiles with a twinkle in his Latin eyes. "Last night we brushed our teeth on the top of the Himalayas."

Meanwhile, not far from the Mendez performance, nurses Kathy Ingallinera and Peggy Wolfe, critical-care specialists, report to work and begin to make final preparations for the patient's move to the intensive care unit. They begin where Cheryl Wood finished last night. They check and make ready the sixteen lines, tubes, and drains to be hooked up to the patient as soon as he enters the room in the unit. The drains and lines include everything from the ventilator that breathes for the patient to the abdominal drains, suctions, and chest tubes.

2:45 P.M.

Since the final closing is still an hour away and hooking up will probably consume another hour and half, Joan, Retta, and Janet decide to get something to eat before taking their first look at John. They leave the hospital, walk across Broad Street, Richmond's wide main thoroughfare, pass the Governor's Mansion and the Capitol designed by Thomas Jefferson, and continue to Shockoe Slip at the foot of Capitol Hill for a late lunch. It is a cold, grey day. They dine on clam chowder at Miller's. The luncheon conversation naturally turns to the surgery. They marvel at the extraordinary string of events that fell together to make this moment possible.

3:15 P.M.

The surgeons are finished closing, and Tom Bowman, the replacement for nurse anesthetist John Beeston, is in the midst of cleaning the patient of all the tape the anesthesiology team used. Bowman is busily cutting away tape so he can present the MRICU nurses with a cleaned-up patient, ready for the insertion of all the drains and lines in intensive care. He turns to the tape on the wrist and begins to cut it away. In the total exhaustion following the all-night operation, however, his colleague John Beeston forgot to tell him about the string on each wrist.

For some inexplicable reason, when he comes to the tape that encircles the lower left arm about three inches above the wrist, Bowman stops cutting and begins peeling. Careful peeling reveals an orange string. Bowman comes within centimeters of cutting off the string, but decides to leave it on because it had apparently been so carefully taped down by Beeston, who had remembered the strings from the transplant meeting. Bowman repeats the process with the right arm. The strings have now survived eight hours of surgery in Bangkok and eighteen in Richmond. Nurse Kathy Ingallinera, upon arriving in the OR from the ICU, immediately notices the strings and remembers to treat them with respect.

3:35 P.M.

The doors to OR 15 swing open and Bowman, Shribman, Wolfe, Ingallinera, and Posner leave the operating room with their patient. It is five minutes and eighteen hours after he first entered the room. He leaves with a new liver and five complete body refills of blood. Another man's liver and the blood donations of over two hundred separate individuals have combined with technology and the skills of an enormous staff to preserve a life. It's a miracle by any definition of the word.

3:45 P.M.

The scene in the room at the MRICU is a madhouse of frantic kinetic activity, as if the transplant has suddenly uncovered and released a perpetual motion machine. There is hardly enough space for everyone as the room fills with nurses, technicians, and doctors who are rushing around, yelling, intent on their own particular jobs. Posner screams, "Hook this drain," and the nurses wish he would just leave and let them do their job. Surgeons are always touchy; their egos bruise easily. After all, these surgeons have just saved a life. How dare a nurse—or, for that matter, any other mortal—interfere with their wishes? It's a difficult adjustment as they find themselves in a medical unit in which they are no longer number-one. They have a difficult time adjusting in this immediate post-op period.

Nurses Wolfe and Ingallinera, like two well-trained athletes in the big game, jump to their assigned duties as soon as their patient enters the room. Technicians, surgeons, and nurses work frantically to prepare the patient carefully, so every possible bodily function can be monitored and tracked. One line in the jugular enables the nurses to draw blood every five minutes for a host of tests. Ingallinera is running through a checklist of sixteen separate items, from connecting the cardiac monitor and ventilator to assessing airway ventilation and perfusion, checking all dressings for bleeding, and keeping the necessary documentation. Wolfe goes through her checklist of nineteen separate tasks, from connecting five more drains, tubes, and suctions to seven different laboratory tests, as well as measuring all intake and output. They work nonstop for over an hour, hooking their patient to the machines that are his life. In addition, they are anxious to clean the patient and get him looking "a little more like a human" before the family comes back to see him.

Settled into the MRICU, the transplant patient looks like an astronaut in space tethered to his spaceship.

4:30 P.M.

Retta, Joan, and Janet return from lunch and are floored at the scene that greets them in the MRICU. Six monitoring machines fill up one whole wall of the room—it looks like the sound system for a Grateful Dead concert. The whole eerie setting resembles a science fiction movie.

Joan peers through the window, thinking, *My God what is technology doing to man? We're making vegetables out of mankind.*

6:00 P.M.

Janet reaches her home and calls friends to describe the eerie scene at MCV. "It was the most incredible thing I have ever witnessed. Everybody was doing something. They were hooking John up to monitors and he had tubes coming out of him everywhere. Every once in a while there would be a beep-beep-beep-beep, and we would hold our breath, but it was just like normal for the nurses. Incredibly, there was never any feeling of alarm or anything, no time when they didn't know exactly what sound went to what monitor.

"They were all just working, and each of them had something to do. It was scary, noises and sounds. For the first time it seemed real. It was just beyond belief. They have reduced a human being to a machine. I had never seen so many tubes. It was like John was just a small part of it, and the machines were doing it all. John would have been excited by the whole thing. I can't wait to tell him."

Retta is now at home calling many people: Ray Wallace, who had headed the fundraising drive; family and friends in this country and in Thailand.

Joan is very disturbed and talks to Jay. "John has all that apparatus to keep him alive. I am bothered by what man is doing to mankind."

She expresses the fears of many that modern medicine, in some kind of strange and perverse way, is degrading humanity. "On the other hand," she asks somewhat rhetorically, "is it something I should be uplifted by? Or is it going against the wishes of God?

"At first when I saw John and the machines and the reduction of a human being to a machine, I couldn't resolve it," she confesses. "I couldn't separate my thoughts. But now I feel it was kind of like putting mankind up on a pedestal—Gee, look what we can do to save a life. But," she continues, "if I had to go through what John has gone through, I don't think I could. I wonder if John himself would have done it if he had known all this."

Jay replies firmly, "He really hasn't been through anything yet compared to what's in store for him. The ordeal is just beginning. I know you're excited about the amazing events of the day, but this is only a beginning. It's premature to say his life has been saved. He's got too much ahead of him."

As a doctor, Jay instinctively understood that nonmedical people always tend to think everything is over with an operation. The public focuses on the day of the operation and forgets the dangers inherent in post-surgical recovery. He was only reminding Joan of what all doctors know, and what the transplant team was especially careful to explain to all potential transplant patients: the trouble only really begins for the transplant patient once the surgery is over.

Jay's conversation with Joan mirrored what Mendez reminded everyone of so many times during the transplant evaluation process. As usual, the surgeon's words were as colorful as they were riveting: "When an orthopedic surgeon finishes, ninety-eight percent of his worries are over. He has put the bones together. But it's all different for transplant surgeons. From the moment we close the skin, we start worrying, because that's when infection and rejection begin. And then, of course, there's the whole set of problems that can result from the inability of the body to stand the immunosuppressant agent, cyclosporine. It can cause mental confusion and serious challenges to the metabolic system [which includes all the physical and chemical processes in the body that change food and other nutriments into chemicals and energy for the body to sustain life]. When the patient has been severely ill for a long period of time, he is weak and cannot fight off many of the complications that are inherent in transplantation. We can never relax with a transplant patient, even years after surgery."

Surgery is a shock to the system and transplant surgery is the greatest shock the body can ever endure. Despite this, however, in the early history of transplant, the actual surgery was not the major cause of problems. Rejection and post-surgical complications caused most of the deaths. But Mendez's historic liver transplant was clearly introducing a significant jeopardy in the surgery itself, because his current patient entered the operation already in a day-long coma, making his chance of surviving the procedure even more remote.

Mendez knew that when and if his patient woke up, the real problems would begin. Infection is an ongoing problem. The transplant patient is mired in an intensive care unit with sixteen separate lines going into him to monitor bodily functions and to keep him alive. All of the lines are avenues for infection at a time when the immune system has been seriously compromised in its ability to fight infection, to keep it from leading the attack on the newly transplanted organ, which it will always regard as a foreign substance assaulting the body. As a result, infection is perhaps a greater killer of transplant patients than rejection itself.

In 1987, transplant was still in its infancy. The drug to control rejection, cyclosporine, which moved transplants out of the experimental stage, was only five years old. There was much doctors still did not know about dosages and about the long-term effects of the drug. There was still a lot they did not understand about post-transplant care.

While Mendez and the MCV doctors had defied the odds and operated successfully after portacaval shunt surgery and a coma, they knew they were about to enter an even more difficult stage because of the complications inherent in a hepatitis B patient. They knew that despite massive blood transfusions and a healthy new liver, hepatitis B never went away. It remained a constant threat despite the new liver. In most cases so far, the hepatitis B virus had destroyed the new liver (to date, none of MCV's hepatitis B patients had lived more than a year). While both Carithers and Mendez believed the clinical evidence did not rule out more tries, nevertheless their viewpoint remained controversial.

There were almost no proven guidelines to follow in post-surgical care. They sailed from the unchartered ocean of transplant surgery to the equally unchartered waters of post-transplant medicine. In addition, they knew portacaval shunt surgery, which alleviated the internal bleeding problems caused by viral cirrhosis in the liver from hepatitis B, meant that the liver's vital function of cleansing the blood was proceeding at a very low level and that an inevitable build-up of toxins followed. They did not understand, in any precise way, the effects of exposing the brain to these toxins over a long term. Clearly brain damage—maybe temporary, probably permanent—could result.

As a physician, Jay understood this and continued to caution Joan. "John's liver did not function properly for years. The portacaval shunt meant that unclean blood was getting to his brain. Who knows what may be done to brain function when a liver is not functioning up to capacity for so long? Remember also he was on the operating table eighteen hours. That long operation might itself have caused some brain damage. We won't know until he wakes up. He may well be a different person. He's going to be confused, and an intensive care unit can be even more confusing. I've read about patients in ICU who reject family and friends. Others are paranoid. I know of a case of man who, while he was in intensive care, continually accused his wife of having an affair."

In Richmond, the same kinds of thoughts were going through Mendez's mind as he relaxed at home and talked over the day with his wife, Sharon. He always worried about his patients, especially after transplant. He was never sure if the nurses and the interns in the intensive care unit fully understood all the problems of a post-transplant patient, whose immune system is severely compromised to prevent rejection. He would "go bananas" if his patients did not get the best care. Many nurses, interns, and medical students had been on the receiving end of his wrath if his patients did not do well. And while survival rates for liver transplant patients had been climbing since the development of the miracle drug cyclosporine, transplantation was in its infancy. So many things could go wrong.

Mendez explained, "Robbins was a long-distance recovery, which meant that the liver was out of the body longer than normal."

"You mean like that baby boy last year?" Sharon interrupted.

"Yes, something like that case," Mendez admitted, as he suddenly became subdued and reflective. Sharon's question forced him to recall the case of a five-year-old boy who was transplanted at the last moment in a procedure that had, like today's, seemingly snatched life from the jaws of death. Although the boy's donated liver had come over 1500 miles, he survived the amazing operation and regained consciousness, but died two weeks later from an out-of-control infection and pneumonia.

"That happens more frequently than I like to think about," the surgeon acknowledged. He reminded Sharon about a 26-year-old-man who survived the operation nicely—the liver functioned perfectly—but who died in the tenth post-operative day from infection. And about the man in his fifties who never recovered his strength after the operation, wore out, and died after a three-month struggle in intensive care.

"Some cases you just never figure out."

Mendez knew that the statistics were encouraging, but not encouraging enough for anything more than extremely cautious optimism. He knew the stats well: of 100 transplant patients, 5% will die in surgery, 10% more will die in the first ten days, and another 5% in a month. Mendez knew that even the 70% who survive the first year will always have problems because they are immunosuppressed, meaning that infections or even simple colds could become fatal. A transplant definitely does not end with surgery. He explained that over and over to patients and families, but no one seemed to get it.

Today's case was even more problematic. Mendez knew conventional statistics might not apply because of hepatitis B. Most centers, in fact, had already stopped transplanting these patients because they rarely survived very long. Often they underwent several transplants, but died anyway. Mendez had defied the odds and gotten his patient off the table alive after a portacaval shunt, hepatitis B, and a coma. But none of MCV's—or, to the staff's knowledge, any other transplant center's— hepatitis B transplants survived very long, though many had actually left the hospital.

The post-operative high was rapidly fading for Mendez. Reality returned. He confessed to Sharon, "We're in for a very difficult time."

In Fredericksburg, Jay continued to explain medical facts to Joan. "That John is alive and did not die in surgery is amazing. He beat tremendous odds, but the odds are still enormous. As his old Yankee hero Yogi Berra would say, 'It ain't over 'til it's over.' And it definitely ain't over yet."

Part III

AWAKENING

LEARNING HOW TO LIVE AGAIN

My hut lies in the middle of a dense forest;
every year the green ivy grows longer.

I have nothing to report to my friends,
If you want to find the meaning,
Stop chasing after so many things.

— Ryoken

1

...a time for silence, a time for speech...

A hole in the world opened up. I fell through and ended up in the Medical Respiratory Intensive Care Unit, a Lewis Carroll Wonderland, where unbirthdays make as much sense as birthdays in its topsy-turvy world.

It's the strange and labyrinthine world of Tolkien's *Lord of the Rings*, inhabited by Hobbits and Gandalf. Tolkien went to Kathmandu, a magical mystery tour at the top of the world, to create his universe. He needn't have gone that far. Any ICU will do. The atmosphere is as mystical, the drugs as plentiful.

It's Las Vegas, a gaudy mix of glitter and showbiz. The people who work there are larger than life. Its dazzle is bigger than reality itself. The ICU casino is twenty-four hours of action with life-and-death stakes. Neon blots out the distinction between night and day. Time passes in an endless continuum, counted as shifts by those working there. Time has no meaning; at best it's segments floating in a void without understandable divisions. You can't tell the difference between 3 p.m. and 3 a.m. Nothing's real.

It's a concentration camp. Your spirit and pride have to be broken in order for you to submit to the regime. The people who tend you are the guards who torment you. The goal is to rob you of your pride, your individuality, your self-respect.

It's like living the contradiction of the Vietnam War. "We had to destroy the village in order to save it."

161

It's like being held hostage. Ultimately you will identify with your captors in the hope that they will be kind to you. Spend some time in an ICU and you'll understand Patty Hearst a lot better.

It's Alcatraz. One doesn't live there; one doesn't rest there; one doesn't recover there. One does time in an ICU.

It's a psycho ward right out of Ken Kesey's *One Flew over the Cuckoo's Nest.* How often I thought I must be in some sort of cuckoo's nest with a bevy of Nurse Racheds.

At first, I was not aware of anything. Machines had turned me into a machine. I was incidental to the process of my own life. Machines do that to you even when you are not aware of them. It is impossible not to wonder whether you are alive or dead when you wake up in such an environment. There is no way you are going to be able to prepare yourself for it. No one can possibly tell you what it feels like. It was another in a long line of events in my life in which the experience and my reaction to it was mine and mine alone. No one else truly knew how I felt. I did not have the expected feelings and thoughts of relief.

I had prepared myself for an enormous high if I survived the transplant surgery, yet I had no memory of surgery. That high, that immense relief, that realization of life extended was not there. *Gosh, I might have died and not known it* was probably my first thought. I was about to begin another experience that was mine alone, that was almost impossible to explain to anyone else.

Confusion remained my constant companion, so I stayed inside my mind, believing the ICU was a place for the terminally ill. I knew no one: family, friends, doctors, nurses. At first, both Mendez and Carithers, reinforced by consults from Psychiatry, believed my disorientation was not out of proportion to the profound insult my body had just undergone, particularly in light of the fact that my end-stage liver disease had lasted three years and that I entered an eighteen-hour operation in coma. That it was taking me a little longer to orient myself was not of great concern to the doctors. The liver continued to function perfectly.

I remained in critical condition for ten days following surgery, which is not unusual for a post-transplant patient. But then things began to go downhill quickly. The twin killers of transplant recipients—pneumonia and infection—combined with cardiac and pulmonary complications to put my life in grave danger. I could no longer breathe on my own, so Mendez summoned a team from anesthesiology to re-insert the tubes for the respirator. I felt deeply betrayed. I prepared to die, because I had been promised no extreme measures would be taken to save my life. (I regarded the breathing machine as an extreme measure.) Carithers explained the course of action to my family, indicating that my condition was beyond the doctors' ability to do anything. He concluded, "Our hope—and it's only a hope—is that he can survive the infection."

I greeted my eleventh post-operative day still on a respirator, with a tube in my trachea, while I tried to fight pneumonia, kidney failure, serious infection, and altered mental states that rendered me nearly comatose. I was tied down to keep me from thrashing about and pulling out lines. The infection was worse and the situation was becoming even more grave.

While I was near death, the frustrated doctors debated. Major doubts as to my survival surfaced among other members of the team. The medical experts were concerned not only about my life, but also about their ability to diagnose. These scientists of medicine didn't know what was causing my downhill slide. They debated potential causes: cyclosporine toxicity, metabolic disorders (inability to process nutrients to sustain the body), organic brain damage. They only knew that they had better do something. And do it quickly. My impending death was bruising their scientific egos.

Twelve days after surgery, Mendez and Carithers confronted a double-bind dilemma: should they lower the anti-rejection medicine, cyclosporine, in order to stimulate the immune system to fight the infection and thereby risk rejection, or continue to guard against rejection and run the risk of death because of an out-of-control opportunistic infection? Such decisions were not anything out of the ordinary for the transplant duo. Difficult choices are around every corner, at all stages of transplant, from initial diagnosis to long-term care. Mendez initially resisted lowering cyclosporine dosage when others thought it was the source of my confusion. Now the demand for the decrease in the drug came because of infection. Although it was not a happy choice, he agreed reluctantly.

I remained in a crisis and on life-support for five weeks. While I survived when many patients with the same kind of complications die, I didn't improve. The encephalopathy (brain damage) placed me near coma. The pleural effusion in my lungs threatened my ability to breathe. Finally, the doctors feared that because of my immunosuppressed status, the rapidly spreading infection in my body could not be stopped. Physicians and technicians from Neurology, Cardiology, and Psychiatry came for consults and naturally ordered batteries of tests. I weathered crisis after crisis. In the midst of this, the nurses still kept a cautious eye on my strings. "He is a Buddhist and on both wrists he has string bracelets that his sister requested never be removed." The doctors continued to debate, test, and hope.

Unaware of the debate, I simply wanted control over my own life. I was tired of reacting, being controlled. I wanted to be in charge of my fate. Sickness and transplant forced me to learn how to take charge of life (and death) in ways I had never before considered. Surviving to this point had meant taking many steps along the road to understanding the puzzle of life and death, and realizing that a return to health is a long, slow, tortuous process.

In the ICU, I became preoccupied with death. I knew I must understand death before I could comprehend life and figure out how to live again. I understood death as a constituent part of life. I knew the impermanence of life—not merely as a theoretical concept, but from facing it directly for years. Death did not hold me—I had long since abandoned my fear of dying. I did not consider death an end, but just a transition point in the wheel of life, birth, death, and rebirth until a kind of deathless state ultimately emerges. I did not fear a final judgment day. I knew death is not the opposite of life. It is natural, the way things are. I was not wrestling with the concept of a second chance at life, but with life itself, and how to get on with it. I knew I must understand death before I could comprehend life and figure out how to live again.

Those who have spent any intense time in spiritual quest know that life, death, deliverance, and rebirth do not exist in a sequential order. The process is circular and ongoing. This becomes evident only when we free ourselves from the entrapment of linear thought and see birth, death, and rebirth as happening many times in our lives. Thus "death" to me meant rebirth in a world of unsatisfactoriness. Our real difficulty comes in expressing this truth. I did not want life where I could not be in control, capable of working out answers to its mysteries. On the other hand, I did not want to die, because I felt I had made some substantial progress in this life, and I wanted a little more time to seek.

Ego reared its head. At first ego startled me. I had sought to suppress it in an effort to remain calm in the face of death during the wait for the transplant. Suddenly, when I realized that I was trying to suppress it here in the ICU, I felt for the first time what my teachers had taught me about suppression and rules—namely that in crisis, a life based on rules and suppression will, like sand, wash away when the storm blows. Peace comes only to those with wisdom—not to those who are merely good rule-followers.

I struggled both for death and for life. For the last three years, death had become my brother, and letting go of it was tough, in much the same way that many men never want to let go of their war experiences or that many hostages identify with their captors. I lived for years right on the edge. There was a kind of perverse excitement in that experience. I was fascinated in a strange way by death itself. I think I enjoyed living near death; it had given my life purpose for some time and I couldn't just let it go because of the transplant. Constantly living with death is a kind of exhilarating experience. I may well have missed the strange kind of high of that proximity when I woke up after the transplant.

I knew I needed time. Winning that time, I turned the ICU into a combat zone, as no one seemed to be able to figure out how to get me to want to live. I became very nasty. I became extremely frustrated by my incremental creep back to health. I did not like to hear that I was getting better when I knew I was not.

At first, the interns in the ICU bore the brunt of my frustration, as I became uncooperative and abusive. "I'm not centered," I protested to the white coat standing above me. I spoke about things the interns did not understand. I was trying to tell the doctor about the Chinese wheelwright who taught that the successful practice of his craft involved a movement of his hands that was neither gentle nor violent. He could not teach this knack to his son nor could his son learn it from the father, because it was a feel that defied instruction. The story formed in my mind as a perfect illustration of my struggle in the ICU. All I could say was "China."

Then I tried to explain to the intern that the balance needed to ride a bicycle was another of those unteachable arts. My explanation didn't register with the doctor. I became frustrated when no one seemed to understand my words and my examples. My desperation mounted as each attempt to illustrate my feelings seemed only to result in more confusion.

With other doctors, I talked about basketball and Michael Jordan. No one understood that the Zen of wheelmaking, bicycle riding, the jump shot, and recovery are all governed by effortless effort, the ability to make the result of an enormous amount of work and dedication look natural and easy. From a Michael Jordan jump shot, haiku, and the Rijoni rock garden in Kyoto to the tea ceremony, a Miró painting, and silent meditation, the best always looks the simplest. Appreciating this Zen of centering and balance means preserving a childlike, beginner's mind. To children all things are possible in their beginner's mind. To live again meant that I needed right concentration to find my beginner's mind, the heart of my childhood—a combination of a Jordan-like concentration and the wheelwright's knack.

I spent most of my time with nurses, who, as the unsung heroes of transplant, are forced to bear the brunt of the patients' frustration and the doctors' short tempers and screams. If you want to know how a patient is doing, ask a nurse. Because they deal with the totality of sickness, they often understand the patient far better than medical doctors and psychiatrists. Perhaps that is because most are women and are less involved in winning and losing than the otherwise masculine-dominated medical profession. I spent time courting, fighting, and—especially at night—philosophizing with the nurses.

First I courted ICU nurse Cheryl Wood, in an attempt to gain my freedom in a personal war against my life-support system, which I hated with a passion because it made me feel totally out of control of my own life. A staff nurse in the MRICU—the tall, willowy, blue-eyed blonde who spoke to me with the gentle magnolia-blossom tones of her Chamblee, Georgia, home—is exactly the kind of woman who always gets my attention. Often when Cheryl was in my room, she would untie my hands and, when she was finished, tie them again. This had been going on for weeks, as I had been slowly courting her. On this occasion, she moved to re-tie my hands, and I motioned to write her a note. "I've been tied for so long, I can't even scratch my face, please untie me. . . I promise I won't touch anything. Please, please, I give you my word."

Her compassion won out over her better judgment and she left me untied. Forty-five minutes later, the normal continuous din of the ICU was pierced by a loud alarm. Cheryl quickly realized that something was wrong with my ventilator. "Mr Robbins, you promised. . . ." Her soft Southern tones gave way to an angry scream. "You set me up!" In quick, angry syllables, she recounted what she saw, that I hadn't just jerked the tube out like most people do, but that I'd carefully untaped it, moved the tape back, squeezed the air from the balloon, and pulled the tube out. She concluded, "It's just like a nurse would do. Now I've got to call Dr. Posner. I'll never trust you again no matter how pathetic you sound."

With another of my ICU nurses, Phyllis Hanson, I engaged in many philosophical discussions. I talked to her at night because I sensed that she understood and, most of all, wasn't judging me as I felt the male doctors were. She grasped that I was struggling with learning how to live again. She appreciated my predicament almost better than anyone else: "He talks to me at night about feeling separated and not being able to be connected with something. I believe John's screams are quite different from other patients'. Others who scream, like 'Lord Jesus what are you doing to me?' seem to be doing it without thought—it's just a kind of learned thing. His screams seem to have more to them. His intellect or intelligence is a part of his spirituality and somehow they are connected.

"His strings tie him to humanity, which he now feels so unconnected with. He cannot connect to anything and his screams are spiritual—not so much a fear of being lonely, but a fear of being alone and unconnected to anything. He is clearly struggling, but it is not a struggle we usually see. It's a mental struggle. His cries at night are not blood-curdling screams of fear—although there are some like that—but more the scream of someone in emotional or intellectual distress. It's like a bit of a wail."

She was right. All along my struggle was mental. As I sought my balance in intensive care, I often used the word "confused" to describe my state of mind. But I realized that it was merely a word, an arbitrary arrangement of marks on a piece of paper or sounds, explaining something I had never known. Finally I realized that a word is a totally inadequate way to convey a feeling. It is like using the word hunger without ever really having been hungry. "Confused" is simply a sound to describe something I had never felt before and hope never to feel again.

My confusion was just another example of my experience that no one else could possibly understand. "Confusion" lasted and lasted, but time stood still and I couldn't figure out why. I searched for words. None came. It was like constantly feeling inappropriate, showing up for a pool party in a tuxedo and then being unable to figure out what was wrong. I was a pinball machine on tilt. I felt like I was speaking a foreign language when I looked at the blank faces staring back at me. My whole world seemed out of phase, except I was never sure who or what was incongruous. It was like living in an eternal present, reinventing the wheel for every task, figuring out my surroundings each day and never getting a grip on reality. Or perhaps it may have been the truest form of reality. Who knows?

I enjoyed my talks with some nurses, but with others, I was nasty and mean. I became infamous in the ICU for my treatment of Sue, a sweet young nurse of Indian descent. I went after her with such a vengeance that she did not want to come into my room. Retta, on one of her visits, witnessed a tirade.

"The nurse beats me, Retta."

"No, she doesn't, John. She's very kind."

"No, she's not, and besides she sneaks me out of here and takes me to brothels. Don't ever let me leave the room with her."

"I won't."

I turned to the nurse, who had entered the room to change some bandages. "Don't do it that way!" I said. "Do it my way; you're hurting me and you enjoy hurting me."

"I'm sorry, Mr. Robbins, but we have to tape this needle down so it won't come out."

"It's not necessary to do it that way."

"I'm really sorry."

Retta tried to apologize, "I'm sorry my brother is being a little difficult."

"Oh, that's all right. This is a stressful time," the abused nurse replied sweetly.

"Do it my way," I yelled.

"I'm sorry, I can't."

"No wonder the British had such trouble with *you* people. Get out of my room, get out of the unit, get out of the hospital, and get out of nursing."

On other visits, Retta heard some of the bizarre tales that the nurses heard on a daily basis:

"How are you feeling, John? You look a little better," she said as she began her visit.

"Oh, Retta, gosh it's good to see you. I've just gotten back."

"What do you mean, John? Where have you been?"

"Tulsa."

"Why did you go to Tulsa?"

"I donated an organ to Oral Roberts."

"That's interesting, John. You don't really like Oral Roberts. Are you sure?"

"Of course I'm sure. I know what I'm doing."

"What did you give him, John?"

"What's down there?"

"Well, let's see now. You've just gotten a new liver."

"Oh, no. I didn't give him my new liver. What else is there?"

"A gall bladder?"

"That's it. I gave him my gall bladder. It didn't work and he died. I left quietly though. No one knows I was there."

"John, you don't have a gall bladder. They took it out in Bangkok."

There are many disturbing aspects of intensive and high-tech medical care that those who have never been through the experience really ever stop to consider. The nonstop care and the machines make you lose faith in yourself, make you believe you are trapped in a hostile world that you can't control. It is profoundly disturbing.

I gleaned now from doctors, interns, some nurses, and even some family members that I was not trying, and that fundamentally my problems were caused by poor motivation. I believed I *was* trying, but I seemed helpless to make anyone believe me. The feelings of those around me became so intolerable that I took what was, for me, a drastic step. I asked for help from a psychologist. I had never thought a person could be talked into mental health and consequently believed psychologists were of questionable value and should be limited to tending rats. I was willing to try now because I was desperate.

Mary Ellen Olbrisch, who had done the psychological evaluation during my pre-transplant days, began spending a lot of time with me, exploring my feelings. I felt helpless and alienated, because I believed that others had concluded I was not trying. Mary Ellen appeared to care and, most important of all, listened in a nonjudgmental way. This lack of judgment was refreshing, because most—but not all—of the medical people I came in contact with weren't so careful in their approach. I was beginning to trust her and believe in psychologists for the first time. I recognized her when she came into my room and felt comfortable with her.

Motivation became an important issue because Carithers wanted to get me out of the ICU. He understood it was clearly no place to get better. He planned to move me to another part of the hospital, the Transplant Unit, where I would need to show more motivation and effort to take responsibility for myself. He was anxious to take that step despite the fact that Cardiology informed him that I had suffered a heart attack (the doctors were not sure when). Nevertheless, by the end of March, my condition had stabilized enough that the doctors considered sending me to the Transplant Unit sometime in April.

The doctors naturally assumed that I would be encouraged by leaving intensive care. Rather than feeling reassured, I thought essential services would be denied to me. Thus the second major problem of ICU care—namely, addiction to the care itself—reared its ugly head. It and loss of faith in oneself are perhaps the two major obstacles facing all patients who spend extended time in an ICU.

Addiction to ICU care can be the most dangerous of all cravings and as difficult to break as any drug dependence. Drug addicts frequently deny or hide their addictions. Likewise, I couldn't tell Carithers that I was "hooked" on the ICU. I chose instead to talk in metaphors to psychologist Mary Ellen Olbrisch. "I don't want to go down. Don't send me to the minors. Don't let them do it to me, Mary Ellen. I'm powerless. Please don't let them give up on me." All I could think of was a sports analogy. The ICU is the majors, the bigtime. Here the accommodations are top-notch, service the very best, travel is first-class, and you've got a future. Once you've been in the bigtime for as long as I have, to be sent down to the minors is the end, the pits. No more first-class travel and accommodations. You have washed-up major leaguers as your managers, seedy hotels, long bus trips, the end.

"I'm scared, Mary Ellen, I'm scared. They're giving up on me and sending me down. I just won't get the care there that I will here. Don't you see, I'm going to the minors. Don't let them send me to the minors, Mary Ellen. You've got to help me. I'm powerless, and they've given up on me. I'm trying, but they just don't understand."

Mary Ellen carefully explained to me that leaving the ICU meant improvement, not abandonment. I was now recovered enough to go to the "floor"—a special unit for transplant patients, where the level of care was certainly above that of a regular section of the hospital.

I thought, *I've always been a verbal person, prided myself on my mind and my verbal abilities, and now I can't put two coherent sentences together. I can't remember anything. It's been a long time since the operation; it can't just be drugs doing this to me. I'm confused. Where am I? What am I doing? What's all this around me?*

I made my last night memorable. Julia, one of my regular nighttime ICU nurses, reported for duty. My wail continued. I rang the bell almost every fifteen minutes:

"I'm leaving, Julia. And I'll die if I leave here."

"I'm scared. Sit with me."

"I don't want to die, Julia."

"I'm confused."

"The nurses in the other units won't take care of me."

"Help me!"

"I can't get it together."

"If I vomit with these tubes in me, I will die."

"Those people are back in the windows again and I'm undergoing another bomb attack."

"Leave me alone."

I was being left to die. Period, end of discussion. I had been hospitalized so long and under medical care for such an extended time that slowly I was beginning to believe that doctors, nurses, hospitals, and drugs were the only things that would cure me. Obviously I needed the best, and now they were about to withdraw it from me. I was begging not to be abandoned. I told myself, *What's the damn use of all this. I'll never be right again. I know I'm crazy because I can't remember things. I'm doing and saying strange things, but I just can't remember. I can't get it together. I know I have definitely lost my center. But I can't explain it. Am I going to live like this for the rest of my life?*

2

...a time for love,
a time for hate...

A fter fifty-three days of nonstop medical attention, I finally left intensive care on April 7, almost two full months after surgery. I immediately suffered intensive-care withdrawal, as the changed surroundings terrified me. I yelled and called the nurses all the time in my first two days on the transplant unit.

The staff held frequent meetings trying to figure out the best course of care to produce improvement in my condition. In early April, Carithers presided at one such meeting, and, after reviewing my medical history, concluded, "We don't understand much of what has happened to John post-operatively. . . . There are many components to his situation that we do not understand in any kind precise physiologic manner."

Mendez was more straightforward, and confided to his surgery associates, "I have serious doubts that he's going to make it."

All I knew was that I was very uncomfortable from a seriously bloated stomach and infections that made all bodily functions a nightmare of excruciating pain. I felt tired all the time and had no strength. In this section of the hospital, I did have to take more responsibility for my own personal care. However, even brushing my teeth or washing my face (though I was still in bed) was an exhausting chore I didn't want to undertake. Eating was entirely too much effort. I expected, and often hoped, that each day would be my last, even though

I was supposedly better now that I was in the transplant unit. This meant I was improving, didn't it?

Perhaps it was medication, perhaps it was depression or dementia, but I got weird again.

"Please give me the parachute."

"Why do you need a parachute?"

"Because I am flying and I need to get off the plane."

I continued my bizarre behavior, confusing time and place. I thought I was back in graduate school and often feared I had missed too many classes and would have to start my doctoral program all over again. I told one nurse, "I died today. It was almost a marvelous victory, but it broke down at night near Chancellorsville. Stonewall Jackson died with me."

At other times my screams of "Help! Help!" brought a nurse running to my room to hear, "Look out, we are under attack, the bombs are taking a terrific toll on us." Moments later, I summoned her to explain, "The Germans have taken over and I am free at last."

The tests to which the staff subjected me did little more than confirm my heart attack and my liver's continued functioning with no signs of rejection. Thus, unable to explain the cause of my physical and mental decline with any kind of physiologic certainty, the doctors concluded that my problems were motivational. If all the medical complications I had suffered in the ICU had not killed me, then clearly I must not be trying, they concluded. But I knew I *was* trying, however I also understood that my effort had to be just right. Unless my effort was just right, I would end up destroying myself.

Long hours in meditation taught me that life and death are really the same thing, and that death is attachment to life. To live this belief, it is necessary to find the right balance between detachment and attachment. I believed that attachment to life was causing me to fear death and therefore to be attached to the struggle against it. I wondered how to fight for life without attaching to the struggle. I feared attachment more than death. I didn't want to die attached to life. I feared that the whole transplant ordeal created a dependence and loss of control. Yet there was, deep in my being, something that made me want to live. But I had to live my own way.

I knew that my whole life had been a search for right effort and right livelihood. Here, in my greatest crisis, my life was still caught up in the dilemma of right effort. It was easy to give up jobs in search of right livelihood. I did that until I realized right livelihood did not depend on vocation, but rather on the way you faced the world. Facing the world requires right effort. Effort is right when it results in understanding. I knew if I failed to reach understanding, life was not worth living.

I realized that the whole dilemma I faced involved *karma*, an idea widely misunderstood in the West, where it is often regarded as merely meaning fate. I didn't think of karma as merely fate, or the result of some action in the past (if you do good, you receive good; if you do bad you will receive bad; the "ye reap what ye sow" teaching of the Bible). The Buddha's teaching of deeds/action/karma was much more subtle and went beyond that of other religions to a teaching of emptiness, a non-making of karma, a non-attachment, a non-doing—that is, living in such a way as not to make an influence on future deeds; to live completely and totally in the present without attachment to the past or the future. I was troubled by a struggle to live to which I might attach and thereby make karma for the future. I had been taught previously, in earlier religious training, that life and death were different. Now I began to understand that life and death were the same, but living and desiring to live were altogether different concepts.

From my days of reading Thoreau to backpacking and whitewater canoe trips, I developed a natural philosophy that could be simply stated as, "This is just the way things are." My meditation master explained that it was also a Buddhist teaching, called *chun nun eng* in Thai. In counterculture vernacular, it may be expressed as "Just chill." It's a concept that recognizes the inherent futility of running against the forces of nature, much as the Buddha taught that the Ganges River slopes to the east and no amount of effort will make it slope to the west. Any attempt to change the course of nature leads to frustration, pain, and suffering. Ignorance is failure to act in conformity with nature and is, therefore, the source of our suffering. If a plant can not live according to its nature, it dies. So, too, does man. We cannot change the slope of the Ganges nor the nature of rocks, trees, and animals. This realization of the natural order of life is the source of true equanimity and the basis of the Buddhist view of life.

In the hospital after the transplant, I often thought of life's endless rhythm of birth, death, and rebirth. I wondered if I had challenged or disrupted the cycle of nature with the transplant. Was my inner being paying me back for the egotism of seeking (apparent) immortality? Perhaps the doctors were now trying to change my nature, and that just wasn't right. Yet I believed that wanting to live was very much a part of man's being.

These feelings caught me by surprise, because I had no idea I would have psychospiritual problems after a transplant. My situation seemed fraught with irony. I asked myself, *Have I complicated my life so I am missing its truth? Did these machines change my nature? Is that why I hated the breathing tube? Have I violated my nature?*

While I debated with myself, the members of the transplant team debated my case at their weekly meetings. As the weeks wore on following my release from the ICU and no one could figure out what to do, the meetings got heated. Mendez remained wedded to the "bad attitude, poorly motivated" explanation. He advocated the "kick in the ass" therapy that had worked with difficult patients before.

"It's all psychological," Mendez chided Mary Ellen Olbrisch, who represented the psychological perspective on the team.

"It most certainly is not, Dr. Mendez," she responds. "You seem to want me just to talk John back into health and that cannot be done. It is not a psychological, but a biological problem. John has serious brain dysfunction of a biological origin. The Chief Psychiatrist on the team, Dr. Levenson, who has been following John since the fifth post-operative day, agrees and has held to this theory almost from his first visits with him in the ICU. We both suggest extensive psychoneurological testing."

These meetings could get testy. They called for all of Carithers' negotiating and compromising skills. Now the unflappable internist tried to sooth the flare-up by summarizing the situation to date. "Throughout the month of April, he has gotten medically better. We started with very genuine concerns about his survival and that immediate crisis seems to have passed. His physical, heart, lung, kidney, and liver functions have all gotten better, but *he's* not any better. He is still effectively non-functional. It seems that a significant part of the problem must be emotional, because if it were physical, he would be dead by now."

He seemed to be siding with Mendez, but, in fact, was following the classical "look at the literature and precedent" approach of medical—as opposed to surgical—training. Internal-medicine doctors follow a systematic approach and do things in a step-by-step way; they rule in and rule out disorders. They are governed by rules and precedent. They don't do something just because it worked before, but because there's proof that it is effective. Surgeons work more anecdotally: this worked once and therefore we are going to do it again. Mendez and Posner: "He's got a bad attitude, so kick him the ass. It's worked before."

Herein was the problem with the multidiscipline approach of the MCV liver transplant program. When the tough decisions had to be made, it was very hard for people who are accustomed to managing medical problems and metabolic disorders, cardiac problems, total body failure problems, to stand back and have a surgeon tell them, "This is what we're going to do and I don't care what you think." As one internist noted, "It's very hard to swallow that pill."

"You're just going to have to swallow that pill," Mendez asserted, not giving an inch. There is one guy in charge and there are a lot people who are around him and that is why many of them say, 'Jerry Mendez doesn't pay attention to me.' Yes, Jerry Mendez listens to you. You have your opinion. But he says, 'No, that will not go,' and people have gone bananas when that has happened. Well, I'm very sorry. I don't do it because of ego. I'm doing it because I think they don't know what they are talking about. I could say 'Go ahead' and I would be so popular they would elect me president. I don't want to run for office. I'm taking care of patients and if I piss people off, it's too bad."

Ann Reid was as confused as anyone. "John seems to be a person who could more or less do anything he put his mind to, and given his strong will, I can't figure out why he hasn't turned around." She cited a progress report from a nurse, Lori Embry, who once again demonstrated that nurses understand patients perhaps better than anyone else: "I don't think he understands the depth of his limitations. He continues to be more inappropriate than most patients. He is not with reality. He's very much alive, but can't get hold of the fact that he's alive. He truly believes he is dead, and he doesn't know what do. Motivation is not a factor at all. A lot of his feelings might go back to his Buddhist faith. He sort of prepared himself to die, and it was hard to get back into his head that he had to live. He's just having a hard time learning how to live."

Mary Ellen Olbrisch noted, "He is capable of a sublime exploration of his feelings, but at the same time needs an approach more subtle than enthusiastic. If we can find this subtle balance I think he will improve.

'Kicking him in the ass' is absolutely the very thing *not* to do. I still also strongly suggest a series of psychophysical tests."

At this point, Bob Carithers, perhaps the team member most skilled in interpersonal relationships, offered a compromise. "Let's send him to North Eight [north wing of the hospital, eighth floor]. It's a ward that will make it necessary for John to take more responsibility for his own care, yet the staff is accustomed to the extreme limitations placed on people by multiple system failures."

Gigi Spicer, the nursing director of the transplant unit; Ann Reid; and Mary Ellen all concurred. Mendez relented and even agreed to Mary Ellen's testing. Carithers cautioned, however, "We must make sure he sees the move to North Eight as positive reinforcement, good news, an indication that he is better. I think the time is right if we move quickly. His biopsy on April 24th once again showed no evidence of rejection. Judy Helfman, the physical therapist, reports he has been walking tentatively with use of a walker for about ten days now. These are the positive signs I think we can use. We've got to be very careful. Remember what happened when we moved him from the ICU."

Thus, my move to North Eight in early May represented the transplant team's effort to force me to take more responsibility for my own cure. The first problem that had to be addressed was my reluctance to eat. I was in a Catch 22 dilemma: I was tired, sick, and discouraged and didn't feel like eating, but I would continue to feel tired, sick, and discouraged if I didn't *start* eating. I felt that I was not eating because all the drugs necessary for a myriad of medical problems kept me confused and disinterested in eating. Carithers, however, told me, "The consensus of the transplant team is that you must take responsibility for getting yourself out of here. You must start eating and taking more responsibility for your own care. We're sending the dietician to help you." I had moments when I did understand Dr. Carithers, but I continued to feel that no one really understood how tired I was and that I had no appetite.

A short time after Carithers' visit, I glanced up and saw a pleasant-looking woman smiling at me. She reminded me of a mother. Her name, Shirley Stover, was on her UVA orange-and-blue-trimmed dietician's uniform.

"I understand that it's up to you and me to get you out of here," she began, by way of introduction.

By now I understood that I had to find the strength to wean myself from the doctors and the experts who had taken over my life. Perhaps I could begin this process with Shirley. I liked her immediately. From the very start, she had an unusual ability to involve me in my own cure. Few people ever walked in my room with that attitude. Most doctors— Carithers being the shining exception—believed they alone could make you well. Shirley began with an attitude of "we've got a job to do." She managed to get off to a positive start with me. For the first time, someone on the medical team communicated clearly to me that I had to cure myself.

"It's been a long time since you've had anything of your own choice to eat. If you could have anything you wanted, what would it be?"

Shirley saw right away from the puzzled look that swept across my face that this natural question was difficult for me. I had been on a restricted diet for so long, I wasn't sure what I liked to eat.

She asked quickly, "How about something special from the cafeteria? We've just started offering fresh-baked croissants."

"That would be nice,"

Shirley left. I really never expected to see her again, since I had succeeded in driving away so many well-intentioned people before her—including several overly enthusiastic chaplains. Much to my surprise, she returned later that afternoon. I was surprised because I realized that she must have stayed beyond her normal shift hours to make the arrangements for my special requests. She told me triumphantly, "John, here are the croissants and butter. Now let's look at the menus and I'll show you some of the special food from the cafeteria that we can have brought up for you." She taught me how to write out menus. I was interested, but wary.

When Shirley returned the next day, she found that I hadn't eaten a thing, but she never accused me of "not eating." She understood that I failed to eat simply because I was not able to—not because I didn't want to. This understanding was an enormous stride, and Shirley's patience and understanding began the long road back to eating. She—unlike many of the arrogant young interns I was to meet—believed me. Shirley's positive approach also led to a vast improvement in my medical condition. My periods of confusion and dementia, which had been becoming shorter and less difficult, were almost ended now. My physical exhaustion, however, continued. Shirley teamed up with some special nurses—Robin Soyars; Frieda Pryor; and Ms. Sydnor, who had earned a special place in my heart with her care and sensitivity—and physical therapist Judy Helfman to make me take more responsibility for my own cure.

I needed an attainable goal, and attending my nephew's wedding in Norfolk, Virginia, at the end of May suddenly occurred to me as a possibility. While I would not be well enough to leave the hospital permanently by then, perhaps if I showed enough improvement, I could get a pass and go to the wedding.

The nurses posted a May calendar on the wall, wrote a big *start* on the twelfth, and penned under it, "19 days." Nineteen days to go before my nephew's wedding. I showed interest in something for the first time in months. The transplant team felt that I should also get out more before going to the wedding, though I was alarmed at the thought of leaving the cocoon of my room and the controlled environment of the hospital.

We went slowly. First, Ann Reid coaxed me to the cafeteria for lunch. Next, Retta took me outside for the first time since a cold wintry February day for an ice cream cone at the Sixth Street Market. Later, Jay came down and drove me around Richmond. Ann Reid, Mary Ellen, and social worker Rick Liverman treated me to lunch at a Chinese restaurant near the hospital.

The trips were a welcome change in routine, but due to the tremendous amount of effort it took me to get ready to go, I didn't enjoy them. The hot weather bothered me. I wasn't real happy but I kept trying, because I wanted to go to the wedding. Ann Reid, a Norfolk native, knew that the church where my nephew was to be married had difficult steps, so Judy Helfman took me to the Physical Therapy room every day to practice climbing stairs.

In the midst of the preparations, Dr. Carithers told me the medical reports were encouraging: the liver biopsies continued to show no rejection, my heart condition had been stable for a month, and I was down to a mere nine medications (from a high of eighteen for three months following transplant). As a result of my slow improvement, he told me the doctors were considering a twofold remedy. First, transfer to Rehabilitation Services for an intensive period of post-operative conditioning and, second, the use of stimulants such as ritalin to deal with depression. I didn't hear him, as I was focused on the wedding. All decisions about the future course of my care were postponed until my return from Norfolk.

Ret picked me up at the hospital on Friday, May 29. She gathered all my medications and all the instructions from the nurses, and we headed down Interstate 64 across the Bay tunnel and into the naval port city of Norfolk. Being outside the hospital felt strange, but I could not dwell on that very long, because it took such an enormous effort by everyone to get me this far. I attended the rehearsal dinner that night and offered a toast recounting a story from my nephew's childhood.

The next day, after the wedding and reception, Ret took me right back to the hospital. I re-entered my cocoon in the evening, exhausted and aware of the enormous effort that going to the wedding had taken. I really didn't want to go out again.

3

...a time for war,
a time for peace...

R eturning to the hospital, I immediately ran into what I regarded as
a hostile group of social scientists who staff the neuro-psychologi-
cal testing center. I was hauled off through twists and turns into the far
corners of MCV where the psychologists play with their rats and human
lives. I met the psychologist in charge of testing. Even in my seriously
weakened condition, I took an instant dislike to him. He gave me
personality tests.

True or False:
I feel tired a good deal of the time.
I like repairing a door latch.
I am not afraid of mice.
I like mannish women.
I pray several times a week.
I used to like to hopscotch.
I am fascinated by fire.
Sexual things disgust me.
I used to have imaginary companions.

I was familiar with these questions and these tests. I had taken them
all before, when my former wife was studying tests and measurement in
graduate school. I knew that the psychologist would use the standard

cookbook approach of personality assessment: reading general characteristics in a book of interpretations according to scales. He wasn't much different from an astrologer and probably not as good. His assessment was astonishingly insightful: "Patient is very concerned about physical health."

One sad result of this whole disastrous incident with the psychologist was my return to a pre-Mary Ellen assessment of psychologists. Except for my friend Sam Simino, who was director of Counseling at the University of North Carolina-Charlotte and a fellow jogger, my opinion of the profession was low. Over the long months of my sickness, though, Mary Ellen had done a wonderful job of reversing that impression. I trusted her, felt she cared and truly took the time to listen and learn something about me. Her associate in measurement destroyed that in a morning. She had to start all over.

When Mary Ellen arrived for her next visit, I complained to her about her colleague. I was, however, growing more interested in other concerns. "What do you think my long-range prospects will be?" Not waiting for an answer, I expressed fears that I wouldn't ever again be able to do much. "I'm not sure I want to live that way, Mary Ellen. What use would I be? This is not a very compassionate society for those who have handicaps, and I am going to have some sort of handicap for the rest of my life. Health insurance is always going to be a problem, and I may never be able to work again."

In addition, for the first time, I expressed to her my concern about the enormous amount of money that had been spent so far in saving my life. I was slowly becoming aware of the very long period I had been in the hospital and the inordinate number of expensive tests that had been conducted on me. I faced the fact that the cost of saving my life might be more than society would be willing to pay for others in the future. Perhaps, I thought, society cannot afford to cure me. It was a prospect I didn't want to face, but I knew it was one that was going to be with me as long as I lived.

Mary Ellen tried to reassure me, but I wasn't mollified. A sickness like mine makes one acutely aware of the contradiction of twentieth-century America. On a one-to-one personal level, our society shows exceptional kindness, but on an impersonal and institutional level, it may be the cruelest in the industrialized world. My personal history of transplant bears witness to this. Enormous personal kindness saved me, but society may relegate me to the trash pile with nothing ever to do again. Americans live in an unacceptable fear of losing everything they have ever worked for because of healthcare costs.

After my bout with the psychologists, Carithers came in to tell me, "Rehab Services has decided to accept you as a patient. We believe your problems are muscular/physical and motivational. We will also be treating you with an anti-depressant drug, ritalin."

"You mean an upper?" I inquired.

"You might call it that."

"I don't like them," I protested. "My problems are not motivational."

Nevertheless, I agreed to go to Rehab. In the elevator on the trip to the basement where Rehab is located, I remarked, "This is like going to Outward Bound." Which meant I approved of the transfer, because I really believe in the Outward Bound philosophy.

Outward Bound is a wilderness survival experience with branches all over the world. In the summer of 1973, I had journeyed to the Minnesota Outward Bound facility. I lived in the beautiful, natural setting of the Boundary Waters Canoe Area and battled steep portages, swamps, rain, cold, mosquitoes, black flies, ropes, rocks, and fear until I learned that I had hidden strengths and weaknesses, that I could find my own way. It was a wonderful sojourn in nature, a life alone—fasting in the wilderness, a three-day solo, and a major expedition through the Quetico wilderness area. I began to understand that while I could not control my environment, I could learn to live more harmoniously with both it and myself.

I was changed after Outward Bound. A year later I was on the road to wander east, searching for life in an intense way—a combination Hermann Hesse and Henry David Thoreau experience. As I tried to recover from the transplant, an Outward Bound-type experience seemed to be a natural way to find my way back to physical and psychic health.

Unfortunately, Rehab was nothing like Outward Bound. As soon as I arrived I felt like I was in a military boot camp. I immediately felt punished rather than rewarded. True to my prediction, I had a disastrous reaction to ritalin. My mind seemed to lose track of my return trip from the wedding, and I believed I was in Norfolk, a city I have never had much affinity for. I felt lost in a mean world of psychologists and social scientists. I could not find any of the nurses who had helped me so much on North Eight. I believed I was forced to share my bathroom with Navy nurses, and at night I would call the nurses to help me board ship so I could help my country!

The Rehab staff of psychologists, doctors, and occupational therapists made their regular visits to see me. I was uninterested and wished they would leave me alone. Surprisingly, one of the psychologists spent time talking to me before coming back to administer tests. His report—"He is philosophically detached from his illness as is consistent with his interest in Buddhism and Existentialism"—indicated that he understood me far better than those who administered the tests, but he never communicated his understanding to me.

I seemed to get medically worse. Dr. Carithers explained, "John, you have some medical problems, and we feel that you had better be back on North Eight. We are not sure if you have hepatitis B, cyclosporine toxicity, or perhaps are in the early stages of rejection. We need to watch you more closely so we can monitor those conditions."

I had lasted four days in Rehab. The ever-watchful nurses sent me back to North Eight with the following warning tacked to my records: "Note: strings on wrist are some sort of Buddhist good luck superstition which patient values highly . . . do not cut these strings off."

Despite Mary Ellen's fears that I might give up, I weathered another crisis. The doctors ruled out hepatitis B, rejection, and drug toxicity, and returned to their original diagnosis of poor motivation and overall physical weakness. Carithers told me, "You need structure and motivation. Your medical emergency is over, so we are sending you back to Rehab."

Trying to remain detached from what was happening and too weak to put up much of a fight, I acquiesced. I didn't have the strength or the words to explain what I felt. I did try an analogy that failed. I told the nurses, "I'm dressed like an adult, but treated like a baby." It was my way of saying, "I'm out of control and before I can get better, I must get control." It was dismissed as another in my long line of weird ravings.

I was forced out of bed in Rehab to eat my meals in the cafeteria for rehab patients. I hated it. I refused to eat. My long-suffering sister was pressed into service to try to make me eat. After spending a day with high school adolescents, she had to drive fifty miles to Richmond and put up with me. She didn't know how to prepare herself for the visit. Would she have to battle me to eat? Combat a deepening depression? Or react to a series of wild stories? Sometimes one visit would encompass all three.

"Retta, did you know that we are surrounded by rapists and drug dealers?" I asked her as we sat in the cafeteria one evening. I complained, "I have nothing in common with these people here, Retta."

"Well, John, pretend you're writing about them, and you have to do an interview," she responded.

"That won't work. See that man over there? I tried to talk to him yesterday, and now he wants to sell me drugs. Drugs are just rampant in here, Retta, and I have to be very careful. Everyone is always trying to sell drugs. You know, what they say about these state institutions is true." I continued. "See that man over there? He raped one of the patients last night. He's done it before, and the nurses are very mad at him."

"John, now you know that's not true."

"Retta, you live on the outside. You just don't know what it's like in here. There are all kinds."

The doctors told Retta to encourage me to eat. She pushed. I resisted. I ended her efforts fairly easily. "Retta," I said, looking straight at her, "let's make our final hours together pleasant. This eating is not important enough to make a fuss. I don't want my last memories of you to be forcing me to do unpleasant things." I could tell by the tears in her eyes that this could be an effective way to avoid things I did not want to do. It worked.

The work of the Rehab Unit is based on tests, and the results dictate the treatment. I took tests, lots and lots of tests. It seemed to me that in addition to putting up with disagreeable nurses and insolent interns, test-taking was about all I did. Speech pathology, verbal expression, occupational therapy tests, neurophysiological functions tests, MMPI, skills, values and interests. My major impressions were tests and tests:

Count backwards from 100. . .
What is the capital of France. . . ?
Please repeat 6, 8, 3, 2 forwards. . .
Please repeat backwards, 7, 9, 6, 8, 3, 4, 8. . .
Please read this paragraph and then tell me the story . . .
Look at these pictures and put them in the right order. . .

Name words that begin with N. . .
Remember Shoe, Dog, Box, Dress, Woman. . .

And, of course, the 566 true-false questions:
I have a good appetite. . .
I am bothered by acid stomach several times a week. . .
At times I feel like smashing things. . .
When I am with people, I am bothered by hearing very weird things. . .
I like poetry. . .
I have never felt better in my life than I do now. . .

The doctors and nurses in Rehab seemed to leave me out of my own cure. In addition, it seemed to me that the psychologists and therapists were trying to get me to do something I just would not accept: learn to live as a person with severe limitations. The implication that I was not in charge of my life sent me into a severe reversal from the progress I had made that enabled me to become strong enough to return to Rehab.

The people I dealt with in Rehab did not have the background to grasp the spiritual nature of my problem nor the philosophical outlook to give patients the time to work out their own solutions. In a real sense, they lacked confidence in the individual's ability to effect his own cure. They shut me out and I went backwards. I stopped eating. I got worse, and for the first time, I was really physically uncomfortable. The doctors could not regulate my fluids. I swelled up and thought I was going to explode. I felt like the man in Monty Python's *Meaning of Life* who ate and ate until he burst. I expected to blow up at any moment. I lay on my side in the fetal position, held on to my bed rails, and refused to move. At other times I felt like one of those drinking water dispensers that has a big jug of water on top. When you press the button for a drink, a great gurgling and bubbling goes on inside the jug. I seemed to be a gurgling, bubbling water jug all the time. I called the nurses frequently. They made me feel that I was really bad for being sick. A group of interns was convinced I was spoiled and demanding special attention. I got to the point where I trusted no one and hated almost everyone associated with Rehab.

As time wore on, I got worse. I hallucinated more and more. Stories I told became stranger and my visions became more weird. I so frequently saw things that others told me were not there that I lost the ability to distinguish the real from the imagined. Life was an unrelated series of events, much as it had been in the ICU. But now it was much worse, because I was never sure what was imagined and what was real. As a result, my whole grip on reality let go. It was not an altered state of consciousness like an acid trip, but it seemed close to what I had read in Castaneda. I saw crows and birds and nonexistent people. I didn't know where I was. I had never felt like that before. It clearly was not the kind of feeling one gets on acid or other mind-altering drugs. I feared the feeling and wanted to get away from it. I hoped I would wake up and it would all disappear. It didn't. I hated to wake up, so I kept my eyes closed. In the meantime, my medical condition worsened.

Mendez came to see me and looked alarmed. Later, he complained to Carithers, "Bob, Bob. Have you seen John? He looks like he is going to die tomorrow. Obviously these guys are not doing the best for him. He has regressed about two thousand light years. He looks terrible. That's a hell of a place to send somebody."

In mid-June, the staff at Rehab scheduled a family conference, and Retta drove to Richmond to meet with the doctors. I was wheeled into the room and discussed as if I were a thing. The therapist told Retta, as one would tell the mother of a retarded child, "He is showing interest in his project. In fact, he shows more enthusiasm in this than in any of the tests and other things he has been doing. But I do have to talk loudly and position myself directly in front of his face to maintain his attention span. Otherwise he drools and goes to sleep." Another therapist explained to Retta, "He simply cannot remember two commands in a row, so he must be told only one thing at a time."

Horrified, Retta exclaimed, "Dear God in heaven, what has happened to my brother. He was fine at the wedding and gave intelligent toasts. I don't understand. How does he lose his mind in a liver transplant? Is he ever going to recover?"

"The psychiatrists think the odds are against it," she was told.

They were convinced, after looking at the results of previous psychological testing, that I had suffered permanent brain damage either prior to or during surgery. The immediate problem at hand, however, was to save my life. One of the doctors in Rehab came to visit me at night. He had already been to see me several times during that same day and his nighttime visit led me to believe he was very worried. Since the

Rehab doctors are seldom around in the evening, I shared his concern. I felt the end was near.

He barked out orders and called for tests. Lab results at 8:30 p.m. showed a marked increase in a right pleural effusion. I had a pulmonary edema. My lungs were collapsing. An EKG at 9:15 p.m. showed continuing serious A-fib (rapidly beating heart). My heart and lungs were failing. He appeared worried but calm as he explained, "We're moving you." Once again the ever-watchful nurse attached a note to my transfer order. "Strings on wrist have some sort of good luck significance and are not to come off."

I was moved in the middle of the night. It might as well have been the middle of the day for all I knew. One hundred and twenty-two days after the transplant, I was back where I started, hooked to machines and subjected to nonstop medical care in the Cardiac Intensive Care Unit (CICU). I was into my fifth month in the hospital and, despite a massive effort, nonstop medication, medical care on the cutting edge, and five moves to different units in the hospital, I hadn't left Go. No wonder everyone thought I was depressed.

The admitting note to the ICU described my condition. "On admission, patient was found to be encephalopathic [a degenerative brain disease] secondary to atrial fibrillation [too-rapid heartbeat] and congestive heart failure . . . and markedly depressed. Patient comes with huge volume of medical records." (For example, the list of medications and blood supplies used so far in my case ran to 400 pages. Reports of lab tests alone filled another two volumes.) I was slightly aware of a constant hustle around me. I noticed a counter and realized that this was not my room at Rehab. Perhaps I was somewhere for tests, because I was getting a test of some sort every time I looked up: chest x-ray, echocardiogram, EKG. I just didn't care. My stomach bloating had lessened and, for the moment, I was happy.

Ann Reid came to intensive care to see me and be certain my strings were protected. "Please make sure the cotton strings around his wrist are not cut. They have strong religious significance."

My hallucinations continued. Dr. Levenson, the transplant team's psychiatrist, found me curled up in bed with my eyes tightly closed. My reason: to avoid hallucination-reality confusion. I figured if I kept my eyes closed all the time, everything would be a hallucination. But then what was real after all? "I don't think I'll ever be able to a get a job again. The future is one big darkness. There is no future," I told the doctor.

His assessment: "Depression appears to be the major impediment to progress at present with complications of poor nutrition. Situation is complicated by significant organic brain damage." He told Carithers this major depressive episode accompanied by mild dementia meant that they should consider ECT (electroconvulsive therapy, or as it is more commonly known, Electric Shock Therapy).

I survived the congestive heart failure and rallied. My lungs cleared, but I spent another five days in intensive care because of a rapidly beating heart. When that settled down, the doctors decided to send me back to North Eight—not Rehab. I was relieved. Once again, I told myself that I had to get control and do something for myself before the people killed me with machines and medicine in an attempt to cure me.

My mind flashed back to a conversation with my brother Jay, several days before in Rehab. For the first time I saw his real frustration with me. And I saw love that passed the bounds of mere concern because I was his brother. For the first time in all my sickness, I saw him emotional and angry. I hadn't easily forgotten the experience.

"John," he said, "I've always admired your ability to fight when bad things happened to you. You've always bounced back. You've got to do something now." And then he said angrily, "You're dying because you won't eat."

4

...a time to keep,
a time to cast away...

By the last week in June, I was back in North Eight, and the debate among the doctors continued. Did my screams at the nurses— calling them "narcs"—mean I was permanently brain damaged and would never get better? Psychologist Mary Ellen Olbrisch stuck to her diagnosis of "organic brain damage, complicated by severe depression." On her first visit to me in my new surroundings, she asked me almost casually, "Do you know what the doctors are considering, John?"

"No," I replied and added, "I hope it's not a return to Rehab."

"They are considering shock therapy," she said calmly.

I guarded my reaction, but I was terrified. *There's nothing wrong with me and now they are going to fry my brain.*

The psychiatrist, Dr. Levenson, returned to see me after the Rehab disaster and began his examination, "Count back by seven from one hundred please."

"100, 97, 90, 73, 83, 87, 67."

"What is 67 minus 3?"

"60."

He stuck to his brain-damage assessment and told Carithers, "We'll discuss shock therapy, but there's a high risk of increased confusion."

On the afternoon of Levenson's visit, Carithers stopped in to tell me that I would not be going back to Rehab. "We're going to make our own Rehab Unit here on North Eight for you. Ann Whitman [the nursing director of the Unit] has agreed to give your favorite nurses, Frieda Pryor and Ms. Sydnor, more time to spend with you, and Shirley Stover [the dietician] and Judy Helfman [the physical therapist] will be with you every day." While the doctors debated brain damage, motivation, metabolic disturbance, and depression, a dedicated team surrounded me in an attempt to allow me to heal myself.

Shirley began coming to my room as soon as she arrived at the hospital, to help me start my day. She brought grapefruit juice each morning because it was not available on the room menus, and I liked it to cover the awful taste of the cyclosporine, the drug I took orally every twelve hours to guard against rejection. The physical therapist began twice-daily visits to get me walking again. I ventured out of my room and, on one memorable day, was able to walk to the end of the corridor, perhaps two hundred feet. I was greatly pleased.

As I spent more and more time with these women helping me, Dr. Levenson told Carithers that I was "definitely improved." The psychiatrist began to back off his permanent brain damage theory. "Definitely improved. Overall I think his encephalopathy [brain damage] has represented multiple metabolic insults to an already damaged brain. ECT consideration to be delayed. Stimulants might still be useful, but let's wait."

In the early evening of June 26, Retta arrived for a final visit before leaving for a month-long vacation in England.

"John," she began, "Dr. Carithers said it would be all right for me to leave. He knows how to reach me. He assured me that you're okay."

"I am. I'll be fine," I replied, not meaning a word of it. And I added, "Mary Ellen told me they were considering shock treatment like the *Cuckoo's Nest*. There's nothing wrong with me! Don't let them do it!"

"John, they can't do anything without our permission. But I'm not sure what to do. I'm just going to have to trust Dr. Carithers."

"Yes, I guess that's the best thing to do," I answered feeling control of my life once again slipping away from me. I told Retta about a woman from the chaplain's office who had come to see me that morning. She seemed different, more relaxed than the other chaplains who had visited me. I felt some kind of instant rapport with her. Surprisingly, I remembered her after only one visit, which was unusual for me. I couldn't remember her name, though, and I doubted that she would be back, because I had taken such a toll on so many people who had tried to help.

The day after Retta left, the woman from the chaplain's office walked into my room. "Do you remember me?"

"Yes, but I can't remember your name."

"It's Barbara Marques. I am in a graduate program and I'm doing an internship in the chaplain's office."

"Yes, now I remember."

Barbara arrived in my life as my slow struggle to want to live again was reaching a turning point. She helped with just the right balance of force and acceptance. She brought two posters to brighten my room. One was a scene of Big Sur, rocks and crashing surf in blue tones, with a caption, "Everyone must set his own course and take the rough seas with the calm." The other was a seashell framed in blue on a pink background. The caption said, "All we need is an ear to listen, an eye to behold and a heart to feel." I turned the captions over and over in my mind and was anxious to talk to Barbara about them on her next visit. I eagerly awaited her return.

Perhaps, I thought, *here is someone who might see the sky the same way I do, and understand.* It was strange that those words surfaced from my unconscious, because they recalled a moment in my life when a group of travelers from all over the world happened to gather on Sumatra, in Indonesia, and began wandering the beaches of the Malay Peninsula in a group we called the Alphabets.

One night our journey found us sleeping on a beach under a moonless, star-filled night far from civilization. Since we were only a few degrees north of the equator, I peered intently into the sky hoping to catch my first glimpse of the Southern Cross low on the horizon. A young Englishwoman who had joined us several days before told me as we looked up at the sky, "John, I could never have a relationship with anyone who did not see the sky the same way I do." I nodded agreement, since we were all into "heavy thoughts." I quickly forgot the comment, but it stuck in my mind and my conversations with Barbara now brought that experience back to mind.

It reminded me that my doctors and I see the sky differently. They have divided up the human being and do not see sickness and cure in the same way as I do. Doctor and patient don't see the same sky—or as Thoreau might have put it, they don't hear the same drummer. Dividing the human irreconcilably into mind and body perpetuates an unnatural dualism that prevents us from seeing and healing.

Barbara returned for another visit that afternoon. For the first time with any visitor in over five months, I began a conversation. "Gosh, I love those posters, Barbara. You know Big Sur is one of my favorite places. That part of California is very mystical and strong. Krishnamurti had a retreat at Ojai not far from there. Have you ever read any Krishnamurti? If not, you should. 'The world is you and you are the world.' He says there is no fundamental difference between 'the observer and the observed.' The world is unified and circular—not separate and linear."

I told her of my knowing that the heart and mind are not different. I shared with her my awareness that yes, we *do* need an ear to listen, an eye to behold, and a heart to feel, but that these functions are really all the same in the totality of the human experience. The mind and body are not different, but are the same. Mind must facilitate biological cure. We are not separate from cure, though words, education, and gender-conditioning get in our way of understanding this.

"Remember when Castaneda was surprised at Don Juan's saying the leaf fell up?"

She nodded warmly in the recollection.

"Why was he surprised?" I asked. "Because we are taught with reason that leaves fall down. We only feel with heart, and this is not as good as mind. Right? We can't really believe our heart. Right?"

I could feel myself getting interested in a philosophical discussion for the first time since the beginning of my illness. I was talking about things I believed passionately. I looked at her intensely.

"You certainly understand this, because we are all taught that intuition, a female characteristic, is considered separate from, and not quite as good as, reason, a masculine trait. This is why, with you and other women, Barbara, I can at last talk to someone who understands."

I fell silent for a moment, then spoke of understanding. I noted that "the way of the East is feminine, and Western men rarely ever understand it. Not because they can't, but because society won't let them."

I told Barbara that Dr. Carithers might come closest because he was not afraid of the feminine side of his personality. He valued feelings and nurturing more than do surgeons—the ultimate masculine calling in medicine. Medicine dominated by men sees health in terms of defeating disease.

"Most of the men around here treat me like I am not doing my job, not helping myself get well," I said. "Women doctors, like Dr. Goldsman, physical therapists like Judy Helfman, dieticians like Shirley Stover, and nurses like Ms. Sydnor and Frieda *feel* and, therefore, are effective in ways that men are not. The women understand me."

Barbara was coming almost every day now. My conversations with her suggested to me that I was no longer merely raving, but in fact seeming to make some sense. I felt in control of myself for the first time since the transplant, because verbalization has always helped me clarify my thoughts.

I explained to her the necessity of finding the right balance and right effort. I talked about a similar struggle that I waged with myself in meditation. I told her, "I sat with my legs folded for so many days that I eventually injured my knees. I tried hard. I set goals. But nothing happened. Everything bothered me. The young nens, or novices, were poorly disciplined. Some other monks were mindless and not really serious. The laypeople visiting the monastery were noisy. Ceremonies were stupid and time-consuming. So I went one day to the abbot, Tan Buddhadasa, to air my grievances and be told what to do. He reminded me that we live in the monastery to fight our ego, which is manifested in the things I complained about. He explained that we go to quiet places to prepare for the fight and meditate to prepare to see our ego.

" 'Now is the time for you to fight,' he told me. 'But,' he cautioned me, 'we fight by not fighting and by not attaching to results.' He would not—could not—tell me how to fight. I understood once again that the best teacher does not teach, but only encourages a student to discover for himself. We are in essence our own teachers. He told me what I already knew inside."

I noted to Barbara that in my studies, in my travels, and in the monastery, I always searched for someone to provide the answer. Buddhadasa helped me at last understand that no one could provide the answer for me. He spoke to me in Buddhist terms, saying that I had to walk the path to lose the conceit of *I am*.

"The path exists," he said in conclusion, "but not the man on it." He asked me if I understood. I thought I did. Obviously I did not—my understanding was only intellectual. Perhaps, the transplant experience provided me the opportunity to see if my knowledge could transcend the intellect into an understanding and a kind of wisdom that could let me heal myself.

I had my answer. Now the easiest part: doing it. I had to unify thought and action into a cure. Conversations with Barbara were beginning to show me that I could still be in control. To me, it was all right to live if I could be in control, if I could do what I wanted. I slowly realized that I might be able to achieve the detachment to live a life after death/transplant. Apparently the corner had at last been turned.

By July, I became more aggressive, and in a much different way. I told the new intern, Helene Goldsman, "I'm tired of this hospital routine, Doctor. I'm going to do something about it. Take my feeding tube out." Later that day I explained to Barbara, "This illness is making me dependent and attached, and I don't like it. To create dependence is a non-useful thing."

On the eighth of July, approximately three weeks after my return to North Eight, Dr. Levenson pronounced me "spontaneously improved." That's medical jargon for "we don't know what happened, but he got better." This ended the discussion about brain damage and electric shock therapy. If I had been brain damaged, then against all odds I had simply improved, without anyone's knowing why.

Barbara continued coming to see me almost every day. Some days she read to me from the works of e.e. cummings, a favorite of both of ours. Other days, she introduced me to poets who were new to me, such as the Indian mystic Tagore. I talked to her about haiku. We talked about the music of John Prine, a folk singer we both enjoyed. She brought me tapes of Prine's first two albums, and we listened to his ballads together. We debated Christian and Buddhist ethics and metaphysics—atonement, rebirth, and reincarnation. I talked about my past, my marriage, my friends, family, and, most of all, about many of my students and what we had learned from one another.

In the meantime, my dedicated "rehabilitation" staff of nurses, dieticians, and physical therapists gave me lots of attention as well. Shirley Stover, the dietician on the transplant team, developed a new strategy of dietary goal-setting. She and I counted calories together. We set attainable objectives. "John, do you know that each peanut contains five calories? Let me bring you peanuts to eat. Don't forget butter and all the hidden calories. Do you think you could get up to fifteen hundred calories a day?"

"I think so, Shirley. Do you think they would pull the feeding tube?"

"I'm sure they would."

The feeding tube was last of many lines that were attached to my arm by needles. Ever since the operation (except for the brief trip to my nephew's wedding in Norfolk) I had been continually tethered to devices that delivered medicine, nutrition, glucose, and blood, or connected me to machines that monitored vital functions. By July, my arm resembled the right arm of a junkie because of the many needle punctures. Many of my veins had collapsed, and finding a vein in which to insert a new line was often an excruciatingly painful process.

When I began to walk with some regularity, I still had poles trailing behind containing the monitoring machines and medicine. I could go nowhere—walking in the halls or to the bathroom—without being attached to some device. As I improved, the doctors removed one line after another until I had only one remaining. It delivered nutritional supplements, since I wasn't eating enough. I longed to be totally free of what I regarded as my chains.

I continued courting the intern, Helene Goldsman, by demanding each morning as she entered my room, "Take the tube out!"

"I can't. The attending doctor won't give me permission yet."

"Well, look! Mistakes are made in hospitals every day. Just pull the tube and I'll do so well, all will be okay." I kept up the pressure and became single-minded in my goal to be free of the last of the lines attached to my arm.

Finally, one morning, the young resident responded to my daily demand. "Promise you'll continue to improve your eating if I pull the tube?"

"Absolutely. I promise. Yes! Yes! I want to get on with life. Pull the damn tube." She leaned forward and, in minutes, I was disconnected from my last line. Freedom! I couldn't believe it. I literally jumped out of bed. I could move around without having little monitors on poles trailing me. I was elated. I showered. I felt almost normal. Something simple like walking to the bathroom was no longer a major production.

On Friday, July 10, 1987, one hundred forty-seven days after the transplant, Helene Goldsman disconnected me from my last line. I had gone from a high of sixteen to, in the last month or so, one—and now, at last, none. There was simply no way to express my joy fully. What jumped into my mind were the words from the old spiritual that Martin Luther King often used to close his speeches: "Free at last, Free at last / Thank God Almighty / I'm free at last."

Barbara came to see me after my last line had been withdrawn. I was talkative. She sensed my changed mood and wanted to know why I was suddenly so much better. I explained by telling her two stories that described how I had learned to face the world. I thought they would help explain my improvement.

"One day," I began, "some Thai students asked me to accompany them on a trip to see a beautiful waterfall several hundred kilometers north of Bangkok. I accepted the invitation and immediately saw in my mind a relaxed day swimming and sunning at one of the many wonderful spots in that beautiful country. We had no sooner left the city than we stopped to get something to eat. We got underway again and then seemed to stop immediately for some other side-trip. I thought we were wasting too much time. *We're never going to get to the waterfall, and after all that's the purpose of the trip.* Finally, late in the afternoon, when we reached our destination at last, I exclaimed in disgust, 'But the waterfall is dry! I don't see anything but a little trickle of water. Where's the waterfall? Did you know the waterfall was dry?'

"The students were puzzled at both my attitude and my questions.

" 'Why of course we knew. It only has water during the rainy season, which begins next month,' came the casual reply.

" 'Then why did you come today?' I asked.

"They thought the question strange and just smiled politely.

"That small event had a profound impact on me. Later, upon reflection, I realized the waterfall began for the others the moment the trip got underway. The dry waterfall unlocked the mystery of dualism for me, and I understood that the doing is no different from the achieving, that beginning and ending are not really different. While my companions appreciated the totality of their experience, I missed the day because of my absorption in the goal. I never forgot the lesson of the dry waterfall.

"I learned another lesson—one about patience, detachment, and time—from Acharn Pho, the assistant abbot at my monastery. He never taught me in a formal way, through lectures or discussion, as did the Abbot, Tan Buddhadasa. It was when we shared seemingly menial tasks, and when I least expected it, that I learned wonderful things from this amazing monk.

"Our monastery, Suan Mok, had a tradition called *Wan Gammagorn*, a day before the Buddhist holy day called *Wan Phra*, when the monks devote themselves to work at the monastery. Our task one *Wan Gammagorn* was to build a structure for evening chants to shield us from the rains of the wet season. We gathered at the structure called the *boat* one morning after our meal. I worked that day passing buckets of concrete along the line from the mixer up the plank to the second floor. By chance, I was in the bucket brigade with one of the senior monks, who had been at the monastery for many years.

" 'How long,' I asked naively, 'have you been working on the *boat*?'

" 'Oh, I think it's about fourteen years now, but I'm not really sure,' he replied with absolutely no sense of amazement. He seemed to see nothing unusual in this, and continued working without comment.

"Thinking that fourteen years was just a little long on any such task and with what I regarded as the obvious question already forming in my mind, I slipped beside Acharn Pho on the next work break and gently inquired, 'When's the *boat* going to be finished?'

He looked at me with love and compassion, a look that I knew meant something wonderful was coming. Then he smiled. 'It's finished every day.' "

Barbara grinned and said, "John, absolutely nothing is wrong with your brain. Your physical condition just made it impossible for you to take tests that would have proved you have suffered no brain damage.

"Several days ago, I met with the members of the transplant team and told them you are a very spiritual person and that spirituality was at the heart of your recovery. I explained Buddhism to the doctors and told them they must understand that all of your post-transplant problems have been wrapped up in the spiritual dilemma that the transplant represented—from an unseemly attachment to life to the use of technology to save your life.

"I explained to the team that the entire Eastern perspective is one of detachment, and therefore you must understand it is all right to live again. I told them you need time. I challenged them to come and listen to our discussions of poetry, religion, and music and determine if it is the conversation of a brain-damaged man who needs stimulants and electric shock. John, your spiritual sense is one of the strongest I have ever felt. Perhaps they should hear the stories you told me today, though I am not sure they would understand."

Barbara was right. Her recognition, though more detailed, was essentially the same conclusion that nurses Phyllis Hanson in Intensive Care and Lori Embry in the Transplant Unit had previously recorded in my progress reports. Tired of the battle and totally bored by the hospital routine, I had finally decided it was okay to live. I had reached this point only with aid from a group of extraordinary women. With the hardest part of the work done, the simple part now was finding the strength.

Shirley began nudging me along each morning. She would wake me up early, throw back the curtains, and give me my grapefruit juice. Next she would get my breakfast tray, warm it herself, and bring it in to me. She did that so I could eat earlier and get better spacing between my meals. We spent each breakfast together. She got me special meals from the cafeteria for lunch and tried to come back and sit with me or send a friend to be with me. She even began cooking some food at home for me and bringing it to the hospital.

The nurses helped me devise a new goal: out of the hospital to meet Retta at Dulles Airport in Washington upon her return from England on July 30. I was inspired but exhausted when I thought about the effort that would take.

One of my favorite nurses, Ms. Sydnor, established a daily regime for me that I had to follow. She would awaken me to prepare for Shirley. I was supposed to wash my face, brush my teeth, and comb my hair. Preparation was so difficult that on many mornings I just wanted to sleep rather than perform the simple, basic tasks of living. Often Ms. Sydnor and I would strike a deal. "Wash your face and brush your teeth," she told me. "You're supposed to brush your hair yourself, but it's so pretty I'm going to brush it myself." Then Shirley would arrive with my breakfast and sit with me, while Ms. Sydnor attended to other patients. I would have my walk, rest, lunch, afternoon visit from Barbara, and physical therapy with Judy. The staff had put together a stable schedule for me that I understood.

I achieved my goal. Almost. Although I had been discharged from the hospital six days earlier, one hundred sixty-one days after transplant surgery, I didn't make it to Dulles Airport to greet Retta on her return from England. I waited at Jay's home while a friend met Retta's plane and brought her to Jay's, "so the family could discuss my condition." Before the conversation began, I emerged from the back room.

"John, what happened?" my sister screamed, in amazement and delight. I tried to explain to her what I had discussed with Barbara. The answer was as simple as it was complex and puzzling: a core of people around me—family, friends, and some extraordinarily dedicated health professionals—never gave up. They kept trying and finally so did I.

The observations of nurses from the ICU to the Transplant Ward and of Barbara Marques in the last month of my hospitalization all pointed to spiritual concerns. They were right. The physical complications were easier to face than the inner task I faced after transplant surgery: learning how to live again. That took a long time. But eventually, by mid-June, I did begin to figure out how to live, and in long conversations with Barbara Marques examined my ideas.

There were certainly other facts that might help account for my slow recovery. Perhaps I was simply too high-risk a patient after all, and really should not have been offered a transplant. (Most centers stopped doing hepatitis B transplants for at least four or five years after I had mine. By 1997, I was MCV's only hepatitis B patient from the early years still alive.) Perhaps the long wait coupled with the portacaval shunt deprived my body and my brain of the essential liver function of detoxification and debilitated me to such a great degree that my recovery took much longer then normal.

As I re-emerged cautiously into the world, I regarded the transplant experience as neither a second chance at life nor a new life. There are, I believe, several reasons I came to this conclusion. First, I spent three long years in and out of hospitals with end-stage liver disease, thereby making it hard for me to understand that I had a new life after transplant. Second, I began the operation in coma and spent such a long time trying to recover afterward that a sudden realization of "new life" never took hold. Third, I knew from the difficulty I had in arranging the transplant that life after transplant was going to be difficult, because I lived in a country with no national health care and I also knew that I could never buy the necessary insurance in a profit-driven healthcare system. And finally, and in my mind the most important factor, my philosophical predilection for Buddhism and existentialism kept me detached from the whole ordeal—which I believe was an essential ingredient in my three-year survival prior to transplant—and thereby rendered a "second chance at life" meaningless.

I believe I was given a chance to *continue* a life. That's a great gift and all I really wanted. As a result, in my case there is no ending to transplant because it will be a central factor in the rest of my life. But then, of course, that is consistent with my belief that there can be no ending in a world of impermanence. In the truest sense, there can be no ending or beginning in a circular world of impermanence. After a life-threatening experience, one never has a *new* life, but one is called upon to figure out how to live in a world in which impermanence is more than a theoretical concept. After transplant, it becomes a daily reality. Attachment to a new birth, a new life, in my judgment will only result in disillusionment or frustration.

Perhaps Mary Ellen Olbrisch's last entry in my progress reports said all that can be said about my recovery from transplant surgery or about recovery from any life-threatening illness—or, for that matter, about any of life's decisions: "seems ready to go on with his life."

What more could anyone want?

Beginnings

Suppose you ask God for a miracle and God says yes, very well.
How do you live the rest of your life?
Walker Percy, *Love in the Ruins*

L ife is complete only by examining its ending. When my meditations on death went from the theoretical as a monk to the real as transplant patient, I understood more clearly the philosophy involved in Walker Percy's question. For a long time I had believed that endings and beginnings are really the same thing. Now I came to realize that a life cannot be lived until it has feasted on death. If, as Kant suggests, the unlived life is not worth examining, then the life that has dined with death is more vital and alive for the feasting.

Thus, leaving MCV did not represent my overcoming a last obstacle on the road to health. It was just one barrier beyond which were even greater barriers to hurdle. If I learned how to live again in the six long months I spent recovering from the transplant, I soon discovered that this was an easy task compared to the one now before me, namely, how to get on with the rest of my life in a society that punishes people for getting sick and in which catastrophic illness means financial ruin and living without health insurance. That took a lot longer.

The first aspect of getting on with or beginning life after a struggle to preserve it is to realize that your experience is unique, is yours alone. During and after my transplant, I grew weary of hearing "I know how you feel," because no one did. They simply could not. Experience only appears to repeat, but like history, it never does. Historians repeat one another and, in almost every circumstance, people repeat each other. Events don't. Family, friends, doctors, psychologists, and psychiatrists continually encircled me with the best intentions and they empathized, but they did not have the slightest idea what was going through my mind or what it meant to be dying. No other person—not even those who counsel people facing death—has the slightest idea of the unique story of *my* life and my death. *No one knew how I felt.* "My experience is mine and mine alone and can never be yours." Those words of the great Zen master were in my mind when I needed them. True understanding is always there at the right moment. It was there at crucial moments for me as an affirmation of my uniqueness, which allowed me—in long conversations with Barbara Marques—to open the door to wholeness.

Another aspect of beginning to live again after a life-or-death experience is to understand that to fight for life is neither courageous nor heroic. Little courage is involved, because everyone would do the same thing in his or her own way. I get tired of stories praising people who face death bravely and who fight for life as if doing so were some kind of special achievement. It is not! To fight for life is natural. A society that fails to understand death tends to distort, or at best to misunderstand, the natural. Death is death. Life is life. And death is life. Life is death.

Another kind of beginning question arose for me when Dr. Carithers told me, about a year after I left the hospital, I had become the first patient who, in his knowledge, was free of hepatitis B after transplant. It was just another in a long line of miracles—from surviving the wait for surgery, becoming the first successful transplant after a portacaval shunt, living through infection, pneumonia, kidney failure, and heart attack to recovering from brain dysfunction. At last, I wondered, *Why me?*

Ultimately I answered that question the same way I had when I first asked the "why me" question in the early stages of my sickness. Neither sickness nor cure was part of some divine plan or the result of blind fate. They were, as I had learned as a monk, in the words of my teacher, *"chun nun eng."* That's just the way it is. When you make *chun nun eng* part of your life, you remain detached from both sickness and cure. And from life itself. Detached in this sense doesn't mean "apart from," but rather *so much a part of* that you are totally still and at ease to observe. The most detached person is really the most attached person. These concepts are not really opposites, but actually are parts of the same circular process that governs the world. Detaching, I gave myself the time both to prepare for death and to fight for life. Detaching, I gave my mind/spirit the power to heal me. It had to be done my way. That's just the way it is.

Another aspect of beginning for me was trying to help others in the same predicament in which I found myself. I asked myself how I could help, since I had no money.

I could volunteer. I spoke at blood-donor drives and at forums on transplant. I counseled with those considering transplant and sponsored a run at the local YMCA for Organ Donor Awareness Week. Realizing that individual efforts would probably not be enough, I tried to influence public policy. This caused me to sway from the detachment inherent in my philosophy of existentialism and my Buddhist beliefs and resume the political activism I had given up as a by-product of my life in the East. I worked for two terms as a volunteer Legislative Aide to Virginia Senator Bobby Scott, testified in the General Assembly for new organ-donor laws, and joined Senator Al Gore's presidential primary campaign in 1988 (because he was the author of the National Organ Transplant acts and one of the first national politicians to understand the implications and importance of modern technology in American life). When Gore made a campaign appearance in Richmond, I arranged a press conference at MCV, where the senator met transplant recipients and spoke about organ transplantation and the need to make it available to the poor as well as to the wealthy. In appreciation, I gave him my prized Carolina T-shirt that prompted me to decide to fight for life that night in the Emergency Room at Chulalongkorn Hospital in Bangkok. I also won a position as a Gore delegate from Virginia to the National Democratic Convention in Atlanta.

I lobbied state officials for a change in Virginia's policy that denied funding for liver transplants and wrote an article on the subject for the *Virginia Forum*, a publication that provides opinions by qualified experts to newspapers, radio, and TV stations throughout the state. I worked in staff positions, developing strategy and issues for local and state political candidates. I labored to raise money for others who were waiting for liver transplants. The more I tried, the more things stayed the same. Virginia, in 1997, still regarded liver transplants as experimental and refused to provide them to Medicaid recipients. Organ donation rates, unfortunately, have risen only slightly. Thousands of people still die waiting for transplants.

Other aspects of my beginnings were further demonstrations of impermanence. After locating my Thai friend, Noui, who had moved to Australia to work, I told him how much the strings he tied on my wrist that night years ago in Bangkok had meant to me. I told him they had survived the transplant and had been a source of great inspiration for me in the transplant experience. The strings, however, did not make it to the second anniversary of my transplant. I lost them somewhere in New York State in the spring of 1988, while working in the Gore presidential primary campaign. They may be in New York City or Buffalo or Rochester. I don't know where they came off. I just noticed one day that I didn't have them anymore. Once again, I knew that my mentor in the monastery, Tan Mutti, was right when he told me to throw away my notes (read: attachments), and added that if you truly understand, the wisdom will be there when you need it. My strings were there when I needed them.

Once toward the end of my hospital stay, Barbara Marques found that a weekend substitute nurse had cut the strings off and thrown them away by accident. Barbara enlisted the aid of my faithful regular nurse, Frieda Pryor, and they searched through the bag of contaminated waste (disregarding threats to their own health) and found the strings among some bandages. Barbara carefully tied them back together on my wrists, and when I woke from a sound sleep, the strings were there. I needed them, too, as I was in a precarious state then, trying to regain my center in order to get better. I never knew about their near disappearance in the hospital until I was doing research for this book.

Barbara and Frieda preserved the strings when I needed them. In the spring of 1988, however, I didn't need them anymore, and they disappeared. They were there when I needed them, and then they went the way of everything else in this world of impermanence.

The same lesson of impermanence emerged from the amazing medical team that had come together to save my life. I had naturally become attached to these people, but within three years of my surgery, MCV's liver transplant program self-destructed. Ann Reid got married and moved to Florida. Dr. Mendez got mad and went into private practice at Henrico Doctor's Hospital in Richmond. (Gigi Spicer and a number of the transplant unit nurses went with him, including Lori Embry, who had put up with my ravings in the Transplant Unit.) Dr. Carithers moved to Seattle, taking Ann Reid's successor, Ann Whitman, with him to begin the liver transplant program at the University of Washington Hospital. The team was there when I really needed it and has now moved on, once again teaching me that nothing lasts.

Getting on with my life also meant separating from constant medical attention. While there is never an end of careful medical monitoring for a transplant patient, doctors and hospitals are no longer an integral part of my life. In the years since the transplant, I have not had major problems. I haven't even had a serious cold since I got out of the hospital. I went from the problem patient to the star patient. My new doctors have even stopped my yearly liver biopsies, since I have had no trouble. I only go to Richmond twice a year for appointments in the transplant clinic, as well as for liver-function and cyclosporine level tests every six months. Most of my time with the new doctors is spent in trying to persuade them to lower the dosage of my medications and in debating the need for national health insurance. My only major medical problems come from side-effects of cyclorsporine, namely a slight tremor in my right hand and slightly elevated blood pressure.

The most difficult aspect of living after this dramatic event in my life has been the frustration I have experienced in trying to regain control. Because of my transplant, I found myself unable to buy health insurance due to a pre-existing condition (liver disease). In addition, my decision to wander the world meant that I had not established a base of publications necessary to return to university teaching.

I wanted to control my destiny, but circumstances—some of my making and others the result of my medical condition—seemed to thwart my attempts at control. In asking myself how I could gain control over my destiny, my life, I recalled Alan Watts's wonderful little book, *The Wisdom of Insecurity*, in which he observed that only when you realize there is no such thing as security, are you secure. Several years after my transplant I restated this axiom: *Only when you realize that you never control your life, are you truly in control.*

This seeming contradiction at first puzzled me until I realized that my life—almost everyone's life—is a set of contradictions, paradoxes, and love-hate relationships. Careful reading of this book will reveal a whole set of contradictions, paradoxes, and ironies:

- I have complained about a country that lacked a program of national medical insurance, yet it still provided a medical system that saved my life;
- I embraced a philosophical and spiritual tradition that stressed non-ego, yet I engaged in an ego-fed struggle to preserve my life;

- I believed in following the natural course of events, yet I was willing to change the natural course of my life by transplant;
- I ridiculed psychology and counseling, yet two of the most important people in my cure were a psychologist and a counselor;
- I was no longer a professing Christian, yet Christians in churches from Fredericksburg and Richmond to Charlotte rallied to help me;
- And on and on.

In other words the contradictions and inconsistencies in *Strings* come from the fact that it is about life. Life is inconsistent. Life is ironic. Life is contradictory.

Four years after transplant, I moved to take control, even though I knew I had to understand that I could never truly achieve it until I knew there was no such thing as true control. I began by working on the one thing I would have real control over, my own body. I began following the government's "Food Guide Pyramid" for proper diet, and I undertook a program of daily exercise. Once again, I had a lot of help. The director of the local YMCA, John Laffley, played a major role in my rehabilitation. First, he offered me financial help to join the Y and next, tricked me into running again.

After I had worked out with weights and aerobic machines for about six months, I asked John one day, "What's the distance around the gravel track in Pratt Park behind the Y?"

"Half-mile," he responded quickly and surely.

"I think I'll see if I can get around it," I told him proudly.

Later, when I came back, John asked, "How was your run?"

"Difficult. I doubt that I could ever do a mile."

"You already have," he smiled. "That track is a mile long!"

John's trick started me running. I entered races. First, 5K's, then five miles. Finally, I returned to Hampden-Sydney College, my *alma mater*, and finished the annual Alumni 10K. By 1993 I was running about fifteen races a year in Fredericksburg, Washington, and Richmond. I loped along at the back of the pack. I found the community of runners extraordinarily supportive. Even the elite runners in the area began helping me. About twelve of us got together and organized the Fredericksburg Area Running Club (FARC). I was a founding member and was elected first president of the organization.

As I took control of my life through running, I began to find that I could also teach again. The high school in Fredericksburg, James Monroe, seems each year to produce an extraordinary number of bright, aware, inquisitive young people. Several sought me out to discuss Buddhism and alternate lifestyles. We read books together and met to discuss them. Sometimes they would invite me to class to speak to their friends or they would bring them to meet me. After I spoke on Buddhism at the local Unitarian Church, one member asked me to teach her Buddhism. As a result, we formed a reading group with high school students and townspeople. Slowly I realized that I did not have to be in an institution and be labeled a "teacher" in order to teach again.

John Robbins nearly crossed the ultimate finish line in 1987. . . . But eight years later Robbins is alive, living well . . . and in the best shape he can remember at a ripe age of 57. On Sunday he will demonstrate how life's greatest achievements can be accomplished after a major organ transplant when he runs the 26-mile, 385 yard course around Washington at the 20th Annual Marine Corp Marathon.

Michael Sandler, *The Washington Post*
October 19, 1995

When three members of our running club won the team title at the 1994 Marine Corps Marathon, I got bitten by the marathon bug. I found a coach, Debi Bernardes, who continued in the long line of amazing women who have always helped me. A nationally ranked sub-masters runner, Debi took my running seriously and began plotting a training strategy for me. Debi is nurse Ann Reid Priest, psychologist Mary Ellen Olbrisch, and physical therapist Judy Helfman rolled into one. She cajoled me through injuries, made me continue running in the pool while I was in too much pain to run on land, and kept telling me I could do it.

I began my training a year before the marathon by testing myself at longer distances than 10K. First came the Army Ten Miler, the largest ten-mile race in the country, beginning, ironically, (considering my anti-war activities in the same place), at the Pentagon and going across the bridges of Washington. I finished that race and moved up to a half marathon, the Road Running Clubs of America Eastern Regional Half

Marathon Championship at the Hampton, Virginia Coliseum. The race was held on the eighth anniversary of my transplant, Sunday, February 12, 1995.

Debi told the announcer, who calls out the name of the runners as they enter the Coliseum and run down the finishing chute, that I was finishing a half marathon on the eighth anniversary of my transplant. That began a flurry of publicity, resulting in an article in the Washington *Post* two days before my attempt to run the Marine Corps Marathon. In a pre-marathon interview with the reporter, Dr. Mendez supplied some notable lines. "He was as close to dying as you can get without dying. . . . What he has done is slowly rehabilitate himself totally. For a liver transplant patient, who has suffered to the level he did, to run a marathon . . . is truly amazing."

The story in the *Post*, stories in several other area papers, and interviews on radio and TV placed a lot of pressure on me. I felt I had to finish the marathon now that I had said I was going to run it.

I love racing in Washington and running among its monuments, around the Capitol, and down the Mall. Things were going well, but I was getting tired by the time I passed in front of the Air and Space Museum. By mile twenty-two, when I was really tired, I had to cross the 14th Street Bridge in the heat of a fall afternoon. Although the Marine Corps Marathon has an inspirational course throughout our nation's capital, it does not have a great finishing route. There are few spectators along the final miles to cheer you on. It gets very lonely.

Fortunately two members of the running club, Will Crawford, who began running with me at mile eighteen, and Chris Campbell, a four-time finisher of the Boston Marathon who joined me on the Bridge, kept me going with encouragement, Gatorade, and Power Bars. After running for five hours and more than twenty-five miles, I had to negotiate the steep, corkscrew hill in Arlington Cemetery leading to the finish line at the Iwo Jima Memorial. At each turn, I thought I would see the finish line. When I saw a sign reading "26" I thought *Oh wow, it's over. The finish is surely just around the next turn!* It wasn't. And then, suddenly: the Finish Line. I sprinted (or so it seemed) across the grass, flashed under the clock, and the Marine put a Finisher's Medal around my neck. I had become a marathoner.

To show myself I was really back in control, I planned to repeat the feat the following year at the New York City Marathon. My good friend from the running club, Gary Censoplano, made every long (over twenty miles) training run with me and planned to run the entire course from Staten Island to Central Park by my side, even though he normally ran twice as fast as I do. He wanted to help me make a statement about running and the importance of organ donation.

On a cold, windy November day, my slow pace kept Gary running three hours longer than it usually takes him to complete a marathon. He was cold and miserable when we struggled across the finish line at the Tavern on the Green. Nevertheless, a week after the race, Gary wrote me. "Thank you! Thanks for teaching me patience. Thanks for teaching me the true meaning of running. Thanks for great conversation, but I thank you most for your trust and friendship."

What more could I want from a chance to "get on with my life" than words like these?

Strings has taken me from transplant to marathons, from beginnings to beginnings, and taught me that no one ever takes control away from you, without your acquiescence and permission.

A Note of Thanks

How do you say thanks for a life? I've pondered this a long while and concluded that there are no better nor more profound words than simply "Thank you." There are so many people to thank that I cannot list them all. Most know who they are, and I extend my gratitude for their concern and help.

I cannot fail to mention someone I have never met and whose name I do not even know: the young man whose tragic death made it possible for me to continue to live. I have always loved young people, been inspired, nurtured, and enriched by them as students and friends. How ironic that a teenager saved my life. I can imagine nothing worse to befall anyone than to lose a son in the prime of life. To think of others in the midst of a tragedy of this proportion is the measure of a truly generous spirit. To the parents of my donor, who thought of others in the midst of their unspeakable loss, I thank you. For others who may be inspired by this story, please consider signing an organ donor card and talking about your decision with your next of kin.

My life has been enriched by family and friends. People from all stages of my experiences surrounded me with support, prayers, and comfort. Unfortunately that was not enough, because I needed money. Three friends from college days—Lewis Drew, Ray Wallace and Bill Ware—took the leadership, along with Reverend Charles Sydnor and the Vestry of St. George's Episcopal Church in Fredericksburg, in establishing a fund to raise money for my transplant. Over three hundred twenty-five people from all over this country and from Thailand contributed. Friends from my high school, Haverling Central in Bath, New York; college, Hampden-Sydney College in Virginia; and graduate school, Rice University in Houston, Texas, formed the core of my generous supporters. They were joined by friends, fellow activists, and colleagues and students from various institutions where I have taught—the

215

University of North Carolina-Charlotte, Queens College in Charlotte, and Srinakharinwirot Prasarnmitr in Bangkok, Thailand. Lewis Drew, a classmate and now Dean of Students at Hampden-Sydney, spoke to the 1986-87 student body there about the plight of a long ago-graduate. The students responded magnificently with individual contributions, while several fraternities, including my own Theta Chi, held fundraisers and contributed thousands of dollars to the fund. One hundred nine students and members of the college community turned out for a blood drive organized by Lewis's wife, Nellie. To them and all the unnamed others, I offer my gratitude and thanks for their generous spirit.

Finally, I want to thank the medical, nursing, and support staffs of the following hospitals who made the medical miracle possible: St. Louis Hospital, Bangkok, Thailand; Chulalongkorn University Hospital, Bangkok, Thailand; Mary Washington Hospital, Fredericksburg, Virginia; and the Medical College of Virginia Hospitals, Richmond, Virginia.

My ever-faithful, optimistic, cheerful sister, Retta; my brother, Jay, and his wife, Joan; my nephews and their wives, C.J. and Lynne, and Bruce and Jean; along with numerous aunts, uncles, and cousins in the complex structure of a Virginia family that claims close relatives to at least third cousins twice removed, formed the core of a family that loved me back to health.

A Note
on the Writing of Strings

The information for *Strings* was drawn from my own experience, my diary, extensive reading of all my medicals records (over ten volumes at MCV) and interviews with most of the people involved in the story. The "Big Three" of *Strings*, Transplant Coordinator Ann Reid Priest, R.N.; surgeon, Gerardo Mendez-Picon, M.D.; and internist Robert L. Carithers, Jr., M.D., gave unselfishly of their time to talk with me and help me piece together those thirty-six crucial hours of transplant, as did many of the following, who granted me interviews: At **MCV**, John Beeston, R.N.; Betty Cockrell, R.N.; Lori Emery, R.N.; Julia Hanson, R.N.; Kathy Ingallinera, R.N.; Hyung Mo Lee, M.D.; James L. Levenson, M.D.; Rick Liverman; Mary Ellen Olbrisch, Ph.D.; Marc P. Posner, M.D.; Frieda Pryor, L.P.N.; Janice M. Rossi, R.N.; Jerolene Smalls, L.P.N.B.; Evangeline Sydnor, L.P.N.; Anne Stier, B.S.N.; Shirley Stover, R.D.; Jeffrey W. Timby, M.D.; Betsy Torkington, R.N.; Louise Turner Bateman, R.N.; Ann Whitman, B.S.N.; Cheryl Wood, R.N.; at **Mary Washington Hospital**, Marsha McGaffic, R. N.; Karen Nunally, R.N.; Beverly W. Payne, E.M.T.; Elizabeth Pearson, R.N.; Valerie Sherman, R.N.; at **Richmond Metropolitan Blood Services,** Pat Bezak; Russell O. Briere, M.D.; at **Roanoke Valley Organ Procurement Services**, Bill Cunningham; at **Virginia Tissue Bank,** Christy Heindl; Diana L. Mills, R.N.; at **Hawthorne Aviation, Richmond,** Manuel Fornosier, Jr.; Robin W. Purcell; and **family and friends,** Barbara Marques; Janet Payne; C. J. Robbins, III; Joan R. Robbins; Retta B. Robbins; Raymond B. Wallace, Jr.

The writing of this book was made possible because I have, throughout my life, benefited from some marvelous teachers, who helped me learn to think critically, to write clearly, and to explore, challenge, and question. My first lessons in writing and critical reading came at Haverling High School in Bath, New York, from my 8th grade English teacher, Karol Anders, and my junior-year English teacher, Mary Hoffman, who drilled into my head the structure of English grammar and drove me crazy correcting run-on sentences. While in high school, I wrote school news and sports for the local daily newspaper, *The Steuben Advocate,* almost every day. I profited immeasurably from my editor, Wally Page, who taught me about organization and conveying information simply and accurately. Unfortunately my pay was based on the column inch, and I developed a habit of a wordiness and detail that has driven subsequent teachers and editors to distraction.

At Hampden-Sydney College, Willard Bliss's wonderfully structured, delightful, and ever-so-slightly risqué lectures forever hooked me on the study of history and the dramatic appeal of a true story; and Graves Thompson, a Latin scholar, in three years of Latin taught me more about language and words—and a wry sense of humor—than I can ever acknowledge. In graduate school at Rice University, Leonard Marsak opened up the whole new world of intellectual history for me. From him, I learned an appreciation of the French *philosophes*, which led me to the existentialists, which ultimately brought me to Buddhism. Bill Abbot, who was editor of the *Journal of Southern History* during my years at Rice, taught me how to read a book critically and to evaluate and explain its thesis in clear prose. And finally, Barnes Lathrop from the University of Texas, who directed my dissertation while my major professor, Frank Vandiver, was a Harmsworth Professor at Oxford University, England, taught me valuable lessons in meticulous and careful scholarship

The most important group of teachers in my life were my spiritual mentors, who taught me that you cannot teach. They led me to insights and allowed me the space to develop a spiritual system that I believe was fundamental to my survival during the years I spent with strings on my wrists. They are my spiritual fathers: the Venerable Chao Khun Buddhadasa, Acharn Mutti, and Acharn Pho of Wat Suan Mok, Chaiya, Surat Thani, Thailand; the Venerable Chao Khun Banya Nanta of Wat Cholpratan, Bangkok; and Acharn Gowit of Bangkok. All of my fellow monks and the people of Thailand were teachers to me, as I was given the rare opportunity to be a part of a centuries-old Asian cultural and religious tradition. I carried to that Eastern tradition its Western counterpart, American transcendentalism, which I learned from reading the works of a seeker who, like myself, spent years alone in nature, and faced an early death, and who has been an important part of my life since my school days, Henry David Thoreau.

And, of course, my first and most important teachers, my mother and father, taught me values that have been important all my life. But most important, they instilled self-confidence in me and gave me the freedom to do things "my way."

My getting it all on paper was beautifully facilitated by David Baker, who acted as my computer consultant and unlocked the mystery of word processing. He impressed upon me the fact that "computers don't make mistakes, people do."

Friends, too numerous to mention, read the book in its various stages of creation and offered valuable comment. I must mention one reader, though—Emory Thomas, Regents Distinguished Professor of History at the University of Georgia. Emory, a friend since graduate school and an accomplished writer in his own right, read an early draft and urged me to publish the book. He supported and encouraged me at all stages of the writing and publishing process. My appreciation to him extends beyond words.

George Trim, of North Star Publications, was willing to take a chance and publish *Strings*. He was the first person in the publishing field who really understood that *Strings* was not just a book about an illness and an operation, but was a teaching book about life and all its inconsistencies. I thank him for his confidence.

Finally, John Niendorff, of Los Angeles, edited the book with consummate skill. His remarkable eye and deft touch immeasurably strengthened and clarified virtually every page of the book. He taught me a great deal about writing, and I thank him.

Appendix A

INFORMATION ON ORGAN DONATION

A word from John Robbins: In a coordinated effort to reduce the number of Americans who die each year waiting for an organ donation, the Clinton Administration, under the leadership of Vice President Al Gore, Jr., and Secretary of Health and Human Services Donna E. Shalala, launched the National Organ and Tissue Donation Initiative. The material that follows is drawn from publications included in that initiative and provides, as of December 1997, the most up-to-date and complete information on this important topic. As one whose life was saved by organ donation, I congratulate and thank the Administration for this important initiative. I thank my publisher, George Trim of North Star Publications, for allowing me to include the following information and an organ donor card in Strings. *I would also like to thank David R. Baker, Technical Publishing Advisor in the Office of Disease Prevention and Health Promotion, Department of Health and Human Services, for making the information contained in the initiative available to me for inclusion in this book.*

The first organ transplant was performed in 1954 when one kidney was removed from one identical twin and placed in the other. With the use of tissue matching and immunosuppressive techniques, the number of kidney transplants reached 3400 by 1980. By 1983, the immunosuppressant drug *cyclosporine* reduced the threat of organ rejection and made the successful transplantation of organs more common.

The cyclosporine breakthrough created a demand for organs that greatly exceeded the supply. Personal appeals for organs were commonly made by legislators or through the media, resulting in disorganized and inequitable distribution of organs. It became clear that there was a need for organ recovery criteria and a centralized network to match the scarce supply of donated organs with critically ill patients.

The National Organ Transplant Act

In 1984, the National Organ Transplant Act was passed by Congress to address the need for better coordination and distribution of scarce organs. The Act established a national task force to study transplantation issues and a national Organ Procurement and Transplantation Network (OPTN). The OPTN was started in 1986, and a Scientific Registry of Transplant Recipients (SRTR), a data gathering and tracking service on transplants, began operation in late 1987. Both were funded by the Health Resources and Services Administration (HRSA), an agency of the U.S. Department of Health and Human Services, through contracts awarded to the United Network for Organ Sharing (UNOS) in Richmond, VA. UNOS now serves as the umbrella organization for national organ procurement, transplantation, and statistical information.

The Organ Procurement and Transplantation Network

The primary function of the OPTN is to maintain a national computerized list of patients waiting for organ transplants. The OPTN includes organ procurement organizations, transplant centers, tissue typing laboratories, hospitals, and voluntary health organizations, as well as patients, patient families, donors, and donor families. Its purpose is to ensure equitable access to organs for critically ill and medically qualified patients and to guarantee that scarce organs are procured and used safely and efficiently. As of September 1997, more than 55,000 names were registered on the national waiting list for organ transplants; the list grows by approximately 500 monthly.

Matching Donors and Recipients

When patients are accepted for placement on a transplant program's waiting list, they are registered with the OPTN's centralized computer network. The purpose of the network is to match donors and recipients. It is accessible 24 hours a day, 7 days a week, with organ placement specialists always available to answer questions.

Organ Allocation

When the patient's name is added to the list, his or her medical profile is entered and stored in the OPTN computer.

When a donor organ becomes available, each patient in this "pool" is matched by the computer against the donor characteristics.

The computer then generates a list of patients ranked in an order based upon medical and scientific criteria comparing all patients in the pool to that particular donor.

Where possible, organs are allocated to listed patients in the local area first. If no match can be made, organs are then allocated regionally. If no match can be made regionally, organs are offered to the highest ranking patient elsewhere in the United States.

Factors Affecting Ranking

Factors affecting ranking may include tissue match, blood type, length of time on the waiting list, and immune status. In the case of heart, heart-lung, liver, lung, and pancreas transplants, the potential recipient's distance from the donor hospital is also considered. Therefore, *each* donor will generate a differently ranked list of patients.

All ranking and matching processes are carried out without reference to race or gender.

Recipient Selection

After receiving a printout of the waiting list, the organ procurement coordinator contacts the transplant team of surgeons and physicians for selection of a patient using the ranking list. Often the top patient will *not* get the organ because of one of several reasons: (1) the patient has to be available and willing to be transplanted immediately; (2) the patient has to be healthy enough to undergo major surgery; and (3) laboratory tests measuring the compatibility between donor and recipient must show that the recipient will *not* reject the organ. If the top patient is unable to receive the organ, the organ is then offered to the next patient on the list. Once the patient is selected and contacted and all testing is complete, surgery is scheduled and transplantation takes place.

Organ Procurement Organizations

Organ procurement organizations (OPOs) coordinate activities relating to organ procurement in a designated service area. OPOs evaluate potential donors, discuss donation with family members, and arrange for the surgical removal of donated organs. OPOs also are responsible for preserving organs and arranging for their distribution according to national organ-sharing policies established by the OPTN.

Transplantation: How Far We've Come

Through the HRSA-funded OPTN and SRTR, the following have been accomplished:

- A system for equitable organ access has been established. All U.S. transplant centers and organ procurement organizations now follow recipient selection rules.
- The number of transplants has risen from 9178 in 1985 to 20,360 in 1996.
- Through organ recovery improvements, the average number of transplants performed from each deceased donor has increased from 2.7 in 1988 to 3.5 in 1996. The number of deceased donors increased from 4000 to more than 5400.
- There was a total of 20,360 transplants in 1996, including 3400 living donor transplants, mostly of kidneys.
- The OPTN and SRTR now offer a comprehensive, accurate data system for the federal government, researchers, transplant centers, and patients to use for policy-making, research, and general information.

HRSA's Division of Transplantation

Within HRSA, the Division of Transplantation (DOT) in the Office of Special Programs, administers the OPTN and the SRTR. Other DOT activities include:

- Providing technical assistance to the 63 OPOs.
- Working with public and private organizations to promote donation. Such activities include: promoting minority donor awareness; sponsoring national professional meetings such as the *Surgeon General's Workshop on Increasing Donation*; sponsoring the National Donor Recognition Ceremony and National Donor Sabbath; and supporting private sector actions that promote organ donation.

- Serving as a national resource to professional associations, health providers, health insurers, state health departments, and the media about donation and transplantation through special projects, workshops, and educational materials.
- Managing the contract with the National Marrow Donor Program to administer the National Bone Marrow Registry for unrelated donors.

Donating Organs: It's Easier Than You Think

People who donate organs and tissues can help save or enhance the lives of up to 50 individuals. There are more than 55,000 patients waiting for organ transplants today. According to the Uniform Anatomical Gift Act, effective in all 50 states, anyone over the age of 18 can indicate their desire to be an organ donor by signing and carrying a donor card or indicating an intent to donate on a driver's license. The kidney and parts of certain other organs can be transplanted from living donors. *Most importantly, people need to tell their families and physicians that, in the event of their death, they wish to become donors.* Family and friends should be encouraged to donate organs as well. Donor families are not charged for expenses associated with donating a loved one's organs.

For more information on transplants, contact:
UNOS (United Network for Organ Sharing)
1100 Boulders Parkway, Suite 500
Richmond VA 23225-8770

For transplant information, call **(888) TX INFO-1**
For a brochure on organ donation, call **(800) 355-SHARE**
For information via the Internet, see the following:
http://www.transweb.org
http://www.organdonor.gov
http://www.unos.org

How Do You Become a Donor Candidate?

Fill out a donor card (such as the one on the opposite page) and carry it in your wallet. Most states have some way that you can use your driver's license to indicate your wishes to be a donor. Some states have a donor card on the back of the license; others have a place to check or a colored sticker to put on the license.

It is also extremely important that you let your family know that you want to become an organ and tissue donor at the time of your death. Ask family members to sign your donor card as a witness. When you die, your next-of-kin will be asked to give their consent for you to become a donor. It is very important that they know you want to be a donor because that will make it easier for them to follow through on your wishes.

It would also be useful to tell your family physician and your religious leader that you would like to be a donor. And it would be a good idea to tell your attorney and indicate in your will that you wish to be a donor.

Below is a checklist for you to use in making it known that you wish to be a donor.

Donation Checklist

❑ Sign an organ and tissue donor card.
    ___ Ask family members to witness your card.
❑ Carry the card in your wallet.
❑ Indicate your intent to be a donor on your driver's license
    (if applicable).
❑ Discuss your wish to donate with:
    ___ Your family
    ___ Your physician
    ___ Your religious leader
    ___ Your attorney.
❑ Indicate your wish to be a donor in your will.
❑ Encourage others to become donor candidates.

Appendix B

ORGAN DONOR CARDS

(Suggestion: cut these cards out and have them laminated. Carry one with you at all times. Give the other one to your family.)

I want to Share My Life!
Organ/Tissue Donor Card

I wish to donate my organs and tissues and have shared my decision with my family. I wish to give:

☐ any needed organs and tissues   ☐ only the following organs and tissues:

_____

Donor
Signature _____ Date _____

Witness _____

Witness _____
(Carry one card with you at all times and give the other to your family)

I want to Share My Life!
Organ/Tissue Donor Card

I wish to donate my organs and tissues and have shared my decision with my family. I wish to give:

☐ any needed organs and tissues   ☐ only the following organs and tissues:

_____

Donor
Signature _____ Date _____

Witness _____

Witness _____
(Carry one card with you at all times and give the other to your family)

Index

Aaron, Ty, 110, 112, 116, 124, 128
Albert, A. B., 124
"All My Children" (TV show), 73
Alpert, Richard (Ram Dass), 5
Alspaugh, John, 110, 117, 121
American University Alumni Language
    Center (Bangkok), 15
Artist, Willie, 128

Baker, David, 83, 107
Baliles, the Hon. Gerald (Governor of
    Virginia), 57
Baltimore, 37
Bangkok, 9, 12, 13, 21, 24, 26
Barnard, Christiaan, 42, 49
Beeston, John, 110, 112, 116, 121, 124,
    134, 140, 149, 150. *See also*
    Transplant, surgery
Bergman, Peter, 73
Bernardes, Debi, 211
Berra, Yogi, 158
Bezak, Pat, 106, 110, 113, 148
Big Sur, 195
Bowman, Tom, 150, 152
Briere, Russell, 106, 110, 148
Buddhadasa, the Venerable Acharn, 4,
    54, 197
Buddhism, 201
    chun nun eng, 46
    detachment, 206, 207
    Dhammapada, 67
    Pansa, 55
    path, the, 197
    right balance, 197

right effort, 174, 197
Sangha, 16
sunnata, 48
teachings, 4, 56
teachings, "Mindfulness of Death
    Meditation", 14
uphekkha, 48
Vissudhimagga (Path of Purifica-
    tion), 70
zen, 4, 31, 166
Byrd Airport (Richmond), 96, 98, 109,
    139

Campbell, Chris, 212
Camus, Albert, 3
Cardiology, 170
Carithers, Robert L., Jr., M.D., pre-
    transplant care, 33, 38, 48, 52, 62,
    63, 66, 71-73, 75-77; day of
    transplant, 86-88, 96, 110; post-
    transplant care, 163, 176, 178,
    180, 206, 208
Castaneda, Carlos, 5, 196
Casupanan, Bennie, 148
Censoplano, Gary, 213
Chalong, Khun, 26
Chanvit Tanphiphat, 17, 18, 21, 23, 130
Charlotte *News*, 12
Charlotte *Observer*, 53
Chulalongkorn University Hosptial, 11,
    12, 19, 24, 46, 207
    diseases, bleeding, 15
    Emergency Room, 11
    Operating Room, 23

229

If you enjoyed *Strings* . . .

. . . you'll want to read **Amazing Grace:** *The Autobiography of a Survivor*, by Grace Halloran, Ph.D.

Faced with impending blindness due to a genetic disease that threatened both her and her unborn child, the author set out to find a treatment for what conventional medical wisdom said was untreatable and incurable.

Today, over twenty-five years later, Grace Halloran has created the first medically documented, alternative treatment for Macular Degeneration, Retinitis Pigmentosa, and other serious eye disorders. This treatment is currently being studied by the Holistic Health Department of San Francisco State University.

Follow Grace from her experience as a teenager in prison through her hippie days in San Francisco and on to her search for medical knowledge as she adjusts to being a partially sighted single mother, tours Europe giving seminars, is rebuffed by the medical community and finally, triumphantly, successfully treats 114 patients.

This is an inspirational story, full of good humor and powerful drama, a story that continues to unfold even today, as Grace is being regarded with increasing respect by the medical and ophthalmological communities.

"The hymn 'Amazing Grace' has over twenty verses, but the life-story of this extraordinary woman has many more twists and turns than that. It's a must-read for everyone, a truly uplifting, rewarding story."

Jerry Tokofsky
Motion Picture Producer

Amazing Grace: *Autobiography of a Survivor*
Grace Halloran, Ph.D.
ISBN 1-880823-05-5 • $14.95
North Star Publications

Other outstanding books from North Star Publications

SPIRITUALITY
Where Body and Soul Encounter the Sacred
Carl McColman

"*Spirituality* provides multiple doorways of comfort and insight . . . a practical book for personal, professional, and deep interior exploration."
— Angeles Arrien, Ph.D.
Cultural Anthropologist
Author, *The Four-Fold Way* and *Signs of Life*

"Carl McColman writes from within a clear religious tradition, but in a way which is open and accessible to people who are struggling with what they can believe. His book will be of great help to many people."
— Kenneth Leech
Author, *Soul Friend* and *True Prayer*

DANCING IN THE DARK
The Shadow Side of Intimate Relationships
Douglas & Naomi Moseley

"A+✓ [TOP RATING]. This book is not for the faint-hearted, but it is for those who want to take their relationship to a glorious level—and are willing to do the work in the shadows to get there."
— *Marriage Magazine*

"Bravo! Brava! Finally a book with real solutions for real relationships . . . a must-read for individuals, couples, and helping professionals."
— Pat Love, Ed.D.; co-author, *Hot Monogamy*

FISHING BY MOONLIGHT
The Art of Choosing Intimate Partners
Colene Sawyer, Ph.D.

Winner: 1997 Clark Vincent Award from the California Association of Marriage and Family Therapists.

"From healing past pain to preparing for a heathy mate, this book is filled with useful insights."
— John Gray, Ph.D.
Author, *Men Are From Mars, Women Are From Venus*